D0232407

# Contents

| | |
|---|---|
| **Preface** | v |
| **About the authors** | vii |

**Chapter 1   Making the link: personal development plans, post-registration education and practice (PREP) and portfolios**   1

The process of lifelong learning   1
Your personal development plan   2
Using portfolios for appraisal/individual performance review and PREP   3
Demonstrating the standards of your practice   5
Preparing your portfolio   10

**Chapter 2   Practical ways to identify your learning and service needs as part of your portfolio**   15

Setting standards to show that you are competent   15
Identify your learning needs – how you can find out if you need to be better at doing your job   16
Identify your service needs – how you can find out if there are gaps in services or how you deliver care   25
Set priorities: how you match what's needed with what's possible   33

**Chapter 3   Demonstrating common components of good quality healthcare**   35

Consent   35
Collecting data to demonstrate your learning, competence, performance and standards of service delivery: consent   37
Confidentiality   46
Collecting data to demonstrate your learning, competence, performance and standards of service delivery: confidentiality   48
Learning from complaints   51
Collecting data to demonstrate your learning, competence, performance and standards of service delivery: complaints   51

**Chapter 4   Women's health and lifestyle**   55

What issues you should cover   55
Collecting data to demonstrate your learning, competence, performance and standards of service delivery   65

**Chapter 5    Contraception**                          81
    What issues you should cover                         81
    Collecting data to demonstrate your learning, competence,    91
    performance and standards of service delivery

**Chapter 6    Sexually transmitted infections**        101
    What issues you should cover                        101
    Collecting data to demonstrate your learning, competence,   110
    performance and standards of service delivery

**Chapter 7    Managing infertility in primary care**   121
    What issues you should cover                        122
    Collecting data to demonstrate your learning, competence,   128
    performance and standards of service delivery

**Chapter 8    Vaginal bleeding problems in primary care**   141
    What issues you should cover                        141
    Collecting data to demonstrate your learning, competence,   153
    performance and standards of service delivery

**Chapter 9    The menopause**                          163
    What issues you should cover                        163
    Collecting data to demonstrate your learning, competence,   173
    performance and standards of service delivery

**Chapter 10    Teenager-friendly healthcare**          187
    What issues you should cover                        187
    Collecting data to demonstrate your learning, competence,   193
    performance and standards of service delivery

**And finally**                                         203

**Index**                                               205

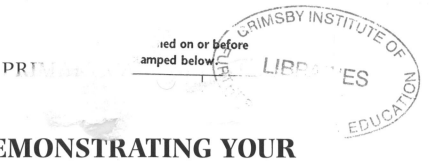

# DEMONSTRATING YOUR CLINICAL COMPETENCE IN WOMEN'S HEALTH

**Pam Campbell**
**Gill Wakley**
**Ruth Chambers**
**and**
**Julian Jenkins**

1857756053

**RADCLIFFE PUBLISHING**
Oxford • San Francisco

**Radcliffe Publishing Ltd**
18 Marcham Road
Abingdon
Oxon OX14 1AA
United Kingdom

**www.radcliffe-oxford.com**
Electronic catalogue and worldwide online ordering facility.

---

British Library Cataloguing in Publication Data

A catalogue record for this book is available from the British Library.

ISBN 1 85775 605 3

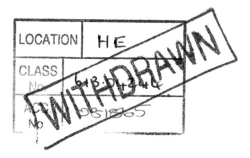
Typeset by Advance Typesetting Ltd, Oxfordshire
Printed and bound by TJ International, Padstow, Cornwall

# Preface

The Nursing and Midwifery Council requires nurses to maintain a professional portfolio.[1] The onus is on individual nurses to decide how they will collect and keep the information that will show that they are clinically competent and that they have taken on board the concept of lifelong learning. Nurses themselves need to decide the nature of the information they collect and retain, in order to have their everyday roles and responsibilities most accurately represented. The National Prescribing Centre[2] along with the Department of Health and professional organisations also advises nurse prescribers to maintain their competency in prescribing using a specific framework.

This book is one of a series that will guide you as a nurse though the process, giving you examples and ideas as to how to document your learning, competence, performance or standards of service delivery. Chapter 1 explains the link between your personal development plans, professional portfolio and individual performance reviews. Learning and service improvements that are integral to your personal development plan are central to the evidence you include in your portfolio. The stages of the evidence cycle that we suggest are reproduced from *The Good Appraisal Toolkit* emphasising the importance of documenting evidence from the learning and practice in your professional portfolio.[3]

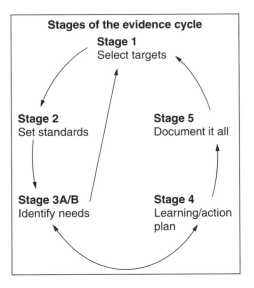

Stage 1 is about setting targets or aspirations for good practice. Stage 2 encourages you, as a nurse, to set standards for the outcomes of what you plan to learn more about, or outcomes relating to you providing a good service in your practice.

Chapter 2 describes a variety of methods to help you to address Stage 3 of the cycle of evidence, to find out what it is you need to learn about or what gaps there are in the way you deliver care as an individual or as a team. This chapter includes a wide variety of methods nurses might use in their everyday work to identify and document these needs. One of the main drivers for striving to improve practice is to benefit individual patients. So it makes sense that we have emphasised the importance of obtaining feedback from patients in this chapter in relation to identifying your learning and service development needs.

Best practice in addressing the giving of informed consent by patients, maintaining confidentiality of patient information and organising responsive complaints processes are all common components of good quality healthcare. Chapter 3 covers these aspects in depth and provides the first example of cycles of evidence for you to consider adopting or adapting for your own circumstances.

The rest of the book consists of seven clinically based chapters that span key topics in women's health. The first part of each chapter covers key issues that are likely to crop up in typical clinical scenarios. The second part of each chapter gives examples of cycles of evidence in a similar format to those in Chapter 3.

Overall, you will probably want to choose three or four cycles of evidence per year. You might choose one or two from Chapter 3 and the rest from clinical areas such as those covered by Chapters 4 to 10. You might like this way of learning and service development so much that you build up a bigger bank of evidence, taking one cycle from each chapter in the same year. Whatever your approach, you will want to keep your cycles of evidence as short and simple as possible, so that the documentation itself is a by-product of the learning and action plans you undertake to improve the service you provide, and does not dominate your time and effort at work.

Other books in the series are based on the same format of the five stages in the cycle of evidence. Book 1 helps nurses and other health professionals to demonstrate that they are competent teachers or trainers, and Books 3, 4 and 5 set out key information and examples of evidence for a wide variety of clinical areas for nurses and other healthcare practitioners.

This approach and style of learning will take a bit of getting used to for many nurses. Until recently, most nurses did not reflect on what they learnt or whether they applied it in practice. They did not protect time for learning and reflection amongst their everyday responsibilities, or target their time and effort on priority topics. Times are changing, and with the introduction of personal development plans and individual performance reviews, nurses are realising that they must take a more professional approach to learning, and document their standards of competence, performance and service delivery. This book helps them to do just that.

**Please note that resources to support this book are provided at http://health.mattersonline.net**

# References

1   www.nmc-uk.org

2   National Prescribing Centre (2003) *Maintaining Competency in Prescribing. An Outline Framework to Help Supplementary Nurse Prescribers* (2e). www.npc.co.uk/nurse_prescribing/pdfs/nurse_update_framework.pdf

3   Chambers R, Tavabie A, Mohanna K and Wakley G (2004) *The Good Appraisal Toolkit.* Radcliffe Publishing, Oxford.

# About the authors

**Pam Campbell** is a principal lecturer in primary care nursing at Staffordshire University. She also facilitates primary care development through a joint appointment with Shropshire and Staffordshire Strategic Health Authority. Her work involves identifying the developmental needs of primary care nurses and providing appropriate education to transform this workforce in line with the NHS Modernisation agenda. Pam has worked in higher education for five years, with particular responsibilities for practice nursing education and nurse prescribing. Before this, she worked in a large general practice for 10 years as an advanced nurse practitioner, practice nurse and health visitor. She maintains some clinical expertise by working in a sexual health clinic once a week. Pam's major interest is in ensuring that continuing professional development for nurses results in changes to the way that care is delivered by providing meaningful education linked to clinical issues.

**Gill Wakley** started in general practice but transferred to community medicine shortly afterwards and then into public health. A desire for increased contact with patients caused a move back into general practice. She has been heavily involved in learning and teaching throughout her career. She was in a training general practice, became an instructing doctor and a regional assessor in family planning, and was until recently a senior clinical lecturer with the Primary Care Department at Keele University. Like Ruth, she has run all types of educational initiatives and activities. A visiting professor at Staffordshire University, she now works as a freelance GP, writer and lecturer.

**Ruth Chambers** has been a GP for more than 20 years and is currently the head of the Stoke-on-Trent Teaching Primary Care Trust programme and professor of primary care development at Staffordshire University. Ruth has worked with the Royal College of General Practitioners to enable GPs to gather evidence about their learning and standards of practice whilst striving to be excellent GPs. Ruth has co-authored a series of books with Gill designed to help readers draw up their own personal development plans or workplace learning plans around key clinical topics.

**Julian Jenkins** has had a longstanding involvement in postgraduate education and many initiatives including novel applications of learning technology. He is a consultant senior lecturer and the clinical director of the Centre for Reproductive Medicine at the University of Bristol (www.ReproMED.co.uk). He is the course director of an innovative MSc course in reproduction and development delivered principally over the Internet (www.ReD-MSc.org.uk) and the chairman of the Obstetrics and Gynaecology education subcommittee for the South West Region (www.swot.org.uk). For many years, he has been involved with the development of evidence-based medicine as a member of the Royal College of Obstetricians and Gynaecologists' Guidelines and Audit Committee and the Menstrual Disorder and Infertility Panel of the Cochrane Collaboration.

# 1

# Making the link: personal development plans, post-registration education and practice (PREP) and portfolios

## The process of lifelong learning

The professional regulatory body for nursing, the Nursing and Midwifery Council (NMC), has stated within the Professional Code of Conduct (2002) that all registered nurses must maintain their professional knowledge and competence.[1] The code states 'you should take part regularly in learning activities that develop your competence and performance'. This means that learning should be lifelong and encompass continuing professional development (CPD). The formal requirements for nurses to re-register state that nurses must meet the post-registration education and practice standards (PREP). This includes completion of 750 hours in practice during the five years before renewal of registration, together with evidence that the nurse has met the professional standards for CPD. This standard comprises a minimum of five days' (or 35 hours') learning activity relevant to the nurse's clinical practice in the three years prior to renewal of professional registration.[2] This requirement is seen as minimal by many nurses who would profess to undertake much more CPD than this in order to keep themselves abreast of current changes in practice. However, many nurses pay little attention to the recording of their CPD activity. This chapter will help you to identify a suitable format for recording learning that occurs in both clinical and educational settings.

Learning involves many steps. It includes the acquisition of information, its retention, the ability to retrieve the information when needed and how to use that information for best practice. Demonstrating your learning involves being able to show the steps you have taken. CPD takes time. It makes sense to utilise the time spent by overlapping learning undertaken to meet your personal and professional needs with that required for the performance of your role in the health service.

All nurses are required to maintain a personal professional portfolio of their learning activity. This is essential to maintain registration with the NMC.[2] Many nurses have drawn up a personal development plan (PDP) that is agreed with their line manager. Some nurses have constructed their PDP in a systematic way and identified the priorities within it, or gathered evidence to demonstrate that what they learnt about was subsequently applied in practice. The NMC does not have a uniform approach to the style of a PDP. Some nurse tutors or managers are content to see that a plan has been drawn up, while others encourage the nurse to develop a systematic approach to identifying and addressing their learning and service needs, in order of importance or urgency.[2]

The new emphasis on lifelong learning for nurses has given the PDP a higher profile. Nurse educationalists view a PDP as a tool to encourage nurses to plan their own learning activities. Managers may view it as a tool that allows quality assurance of the nurse's performance. Nurses, striving to improve the quality of the care that they deliver to patients, may want to use a PDP to guide them on their way, perhaps towards post-registration awards or towards gaining promotion opportunities.

# Your personal development plan

Your PDP will be an integral part of your annual appraisal (sometimes referred to as an individual performance review) and your portfolio that is required by the NMC to demonstrate your fitness to practise as a nurse.

Your initial plan should:

- identify your gaps or weaknesses in knowledge, skills or attitudes
- specify topics for learning as a result of changes: in your role, responsibilities, the organisation in which you work
- link into the learning needs of others in your workplace or team of colleagues
- tie in with the service development priorities of your practice, the primary care organisation (PCO), hospital trust or the NHS as a whole
- describe how you identified your learning needs
- set your learning needs and associated goals in order of importance and urgency
- justify your selection of learning goals
- describe how you will achieve your goals and over what time period
- describe how you will evaluate learning outcomes.[3]

Each year you will continue or revise your PDP. It should demonstrate how you carried out your learning and evaluation plans, show that you have learnt what you set out to do (or why it was modified) and how you applied your new learning in practice. In addition, you will find that you have new priorities and fresh learning needs as circumstances change.

The main task is to capture what you have learnt, in a way that suits you. Then you can look back at what you have done and:

- reflect on it later, to decide to learn more, or to make changes as a result, and identify further needs
- demonstrate to others that you are fit to practise or work through:
  - what you have done
  - what you have learnt
  - what changes you have made as a result
  - the standards of work you have achieved and are maintaining
  - how you monitor your performance at work

- use it to show how your personal learning fits in with the requirements of your practice or the NHS, and other people's personal and professional development plans.

Incorporate all the evidence of your learning into your personal professional profile (PPP). Evidence from this document will be needed if you are asked to take part in the NMC audit, which is designed to ensure that all nurses are complying with the PREP standard. It is up to you how you keep this record of your learning. Examples are:

- *an ongoing learning journal* in which you draw up and describe your plan, record how you determined your needs and prioritised them, report why you attended particular educational meetings or courses and what you got out of them, as well as the continuing cycle of review, making changes and evaluating them
- *an A4 file* with lots of plastic sleeves into which you build up a systematic record of your educational activities in line with your plan
- *a box*: chuck in everything to do with your learning plan as you do it and sort it out into a sensible order every few months with a good review once a year.

# Using portfolios for appraisal/individual performance review and PREP

Appraisal is widely accepted in the NHS as a formative process that should be concerned with the professional development and personal fulfilment of the individual, leading to an improvement in their performance at work. It is a formal structured opportunity whereby the person being appraised has the opportunity to reflect on their work and to consider how their effectiveness might be improved. This positive interpretation of the appraisal process supports the delivery of high-quality patient care and drive to improve clinical standards. Appraisal has been in place in industry, commerce and public sectors for decades. In the NHS, nurses and other health professionals, managers and administrative staff are now all expected to undergo annual appraisals.

Nurses working in the health service should receive an appraisal or individual performance review at least once a year. This appraisal should include two main functions. Firstly, there should be an assessment of fitness to practise in the current role, and secondly there should be a review of the CPD that has taken place and that is needed for the future. This should focus on the needs of the individual together with the needs of the organisation for which the nurse works.

Details of how annual appraisals are structured will vary from one organisation to another, but the educational principles remain the same. The aims are to give nurses an opportunity to discuss and receive regular feedback on their previous and continuing performance, and identify education and development needs.

The United Kingdom Central Council (UKCC) first introduced in 1995 the need to demonstrate that you have undertaken meaningful learning activities, directly related to your nursing role. As the superseding professional body, the NMC has maintained this PREP requirement. When you apply to renew your registration as a nurse every three years, you are required to sign a notification of practice form that includes a declaration that you have met the PREP requirements. This means that your employer may be at liberty to ask to see your PPP that will show the learning activities undertaken and how these have influenced your work. The term portfolio and profile tend to be used synonymously in nursing. A helpful view on distinguishing between the two terms has been given by Rosslyn Brown who views the portfolio as encompassing the development of the individual as a whole (including both personal and professional perspectives) whereas the profile provides a more focused approach to the professional development and may be produced for a more clearly defined audience.[4]

The English National Board (ENB) stipulated that portfolios should be incorporated into pre-registration nursing programmes in 1997.[5] This demonstrates that portfolios are designated as part of the culture of nursing. They should not be viewed simply as a tool for assessing outcomes of courses, but as meaningful documents that provide firm evidence of an individual's journey and progression within nursing. You do not need to set out your portfolio in any specific format. In fact, one of the benefits of using a portfolio is that it allows you to be creative and to produce evidence about your practice in a way that reflects your individual style. However, there are certain elements that should be included. Quinn suggests six main areas: [6]

- factual information: e.g. qualifications, job description, etc
- self-evaluation of professional performance
- action plans/PDP
- documentation of any formal learning undertaken, such as courses attended, etc
- documentation of informal learning, such as reading journal articles that have altered your practice by providing a firm evidence base to follow
- documentation of hours worked between registration periods. This may be particularly important if you do not have a regular contract of employment.

A portfolio will provide evidence that you have complied with the NMC *Code of Professional Conduct* (2002). This clearly states that your professional knowledge must be maintained in the ways given in Box 1.1:[1]

---

**Box 1.1:** Nursing and Midwifery Council requirements for maintaining professional knowledge

- You must keep your knowledge and skills up to date throughout your working life. In particular, you should take part regularly in learning activities that develop your confidence and performance.
- To practise competently, you must possess the knowledge, skills and abilities required for lawful, safe and effective practice without direct supervision. You must acknowledge the limits of your professional competence and only undertake practice and accept responsibilities for those activities in which you are competent.
- If an aspect of practice is beyond your level of competence or outside your area of registration, you must obtain help and supervision from a competent practitioner until you and your employer consider that you have acquired the requisite knowledge and skill.

- You have a duty to facilitate students of nursing and midwifery and others to develop their competence.
- You have a responsibility to deliver care based on current evidence, best practice and, where applicable, validated research when it is available.

Reproduced from: Nursing and Midwifery Council (2002) *Code of Professional Conduct*. NMC, London.[1]

Lifelong learning is a concept that is advocated by the NMC in order to develop professional knowledge and competence, to improve patient care.[7] Lifelong learning can be structured to ensure that learning is meaningful and relevant to your current role. The best way to do this is to incorporate a PDP as a central part of your portfolio. It provides a framework to highlight your learning needs and demonstrates self-awareness and organisation of prioritised learning. Ideally, the PDP should arise from your individual personal review, as this will have utilised both subjective and objective assessments to highlight your developmental needs.

# Demonstrating the standards of your practice

The NMC sets out standards that must be met as part of the duties and responsibilities of nurses in the *Code of Professional Conduct*.[1] These clauses within the code have been drawn up to create expectations for the public relating to the behaviour that they can expect from nurses, and to create a uniform standard of behaviour with which all nurses must comply. A good portfolio should reflect these standards of care wherever possible. For example, confidential information should be protected, so that if your portfolio includes reflective writing there should be no way of identifying specific patients within this. The clauses within the code of conduct are shared values from all the UK healthcare regulatory bodies (*see* Box 1.2).

---

**Box 1.2:**   Clauses to consider when creating a portfolio that relates to clinical care

In caring for patients and clients, you must:

- respect the patient or client as an individual
- obtain consent before you give any treatment or care
- protect confidential information
- co-operate with others in the team
- maintain your professional knowledge and competence
- be trustworthy
- act to identify and minimise risk to patients and clients.

Reproduced from: Nursing and Midwifery Council (2002) *Code of Professional Conduct*. NMC, London.[1]

---

In order to demonstrate that your clinical practice upholds these professional standards, you will need to include evidence within your portfolio. The evidence cycle shown in Figure 1.1 provides a comprehensive model for demonstrating your standards of practice and how you seek to improve them. The stages of the evidence cycle are common to all the various areas of expertise considered in this book and will be followed in each chapter.

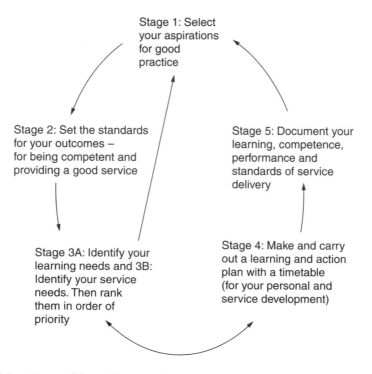

**Figure 1.1:**   Stages of the evidence cycle.

Although the five stages are shown in sequence here, in practice you would expect to move backwards and forwards from stage to stage, because of new information or a modification of your earlier ideas. New information might accrue when research is published which affects your clinical behaviour or standards, or a critical incident or patient complaint might occur which causes you and others to think anew about your standards or the way that services are delivered. The arrows in Figure 1.1 show that you might reset your target or aspirations for good practice having undertaken exercises to identify what you need to learn or determine whether there are gaps in service delivery.

We suggest that you demonstrate your competence in focused areas of your day-to-day work by completing several cycles of evidence drawn from a variety of clinical or other areas each year.

As you start to collate information about this five-stage cycle, discuss any problems about the standards of care or services you are looking at, with colleagues, experts in this area, tutors, etc. You want to develop a wide range and depth of evidence so that you can show that you are competent in your day-to-day general work as well as for any special areas of expertise.

Professional competence is the first area of concern to employers and the public. You should be able to demonstrate that you can maintain a satisfactory standard of clinical care most of the time in your everyday work. Some of the time you will be brilliant, of course! Celebrate those moments. On other occasions, you or others around you will be critical of your performance and feel that you could have done much better. Reflect on those episodes to learn from them.

## Stage 1: Select your aspirations for good practice

By adopting or adapting descriptions of what an 'excellent' nurse should be aiming for, you are defining the standards of practice for which you, as an individual nurse, should be aiming. You may find it easier to define your standards initially in terms of what standards are unacceptable to you. Your standards may be influenced by role models whom you have identified as being particularly skilled in a certain area of practice. It may be helpful to note down these particular qualities to which you aspire. However, it is also useful to note that some practitioners define 'excellence' as being consistently good.[8] You may recognise that this is much harder to achieve (and demonstrate) than sporadic bursts of excellence.

This consistency is a critical factor in considering competence and performance too (*see* page 15). The documents that you collect in your evidence cycles must reflect consistency over time and in different circumstances, for example with various types of patients, or your practice at different times of day. This will show that you have not only performed well on one occasion or for one type of baseline assessment, but also sustained your performance over time and under different conditions.

## Stage 2: Set the standards for your outcomes – for being competent and providing a good service

Outcomes might include:

- the way that learning is applied
- a learnt skill
- a protocol
- a strategy that is implemented
- meeting recommended standards.

The level at which you should be performing depends on your particular field of expertise. Generalist nurses are good at seeing the wider picture, while specialists tend to be expert in a narrow area, so that the level of competence expected for a clinical area will vary depending on the nurse's role and responsibilities. You would not, for example, expect nurse specialists in women's health to be competent at managing patients with cardiac failure (although some of them may be), but you would expect practice nurses to be able to manage a wide variety of conditions, but with limited expertise in certain areas. You would expect both the specialist nurse and the generalist nurse to recognise their 'scope of practice' and to refer to someone with more expertise when necessary.[9]

Other standards include using resources effectively and the record keeping that is an essential tool in clinical care. As a health professional, you need to be accessible and available so that you can provide your services, and make suitable arrangements for handing over care to others. You could incorporate into your standards or outcomes those components specified by universities at a national level as part of their Masters' Frameworks for their postgraduate awards. The Masters' Frameworks consist of eight components that shape the individual postgraduate award programme outcomes and the learning outcomes of the individual modules for the postgraduate awards. The eight components are shown in Box 1.3. You could set out your CPD work in the portfolio you are assembling for revalidation and your annual appraisals in this format. This would help you to document your professional development to date in a form that can be readily 'accredited for prior experiential learning' (APEL) by universities (contact your local universities if you want more information about this process). You might then be given credits for learning against an intended postgraduate award. It would save you from duplicating work as well as speeding your progress through the award.

---

**Box 1.3:**    The eight components of the Masters' Frameworks for postgraduate awards

1   Analysis
2   Problem solving
3   Knowledge and understanding
4   Reflection
5   Communication
6   Learning
7   Application
8   Enquiry

---

If you have information or data about your practice showing that it was substandard or that you were not competent, you might choose to exclude that from your portfolio. However, you will be able to show that you have learnt more by reviewing mistakes or negative episodes. It is better to include everything of relevance, then go on to demonstrate how you addressed the gaps in your performance and made sustained improvements. As highlighted earlier, you will need to protect the confidentiality of patients and colleagues as necessary when you collect data. The NMC will be seeing the contents of your portfolio if it is randomly selected for review. You will probably also submit or share the documentation for job interviews and for your appraisal and maybe use it for reviews within clinical supervision sessions.

## Stage 3: Identify your learning and service needs in your practice or primary care organisation and rank them in order of priority[3]

The type and depth of documentation you need to gather will encompass:

- the context in which you work
- your knowledge and skills in relation to any particular role or responsibility of your current post.

The extent of expertise you should possess will depend on your level of responsibility for a particular function or task. You may be personally responsible for that function or task, or you may contribute to or delegate responsibility for it. Your learning needs should take into account your aspirations for the future too – personal or career development for you, or improvements in the way you deliver care in your practice. Look at Chapter 2 for more ideas on how you will identify your learning or service development needs.

Group and summarise your service development needs from the exercises you have carried out. Grade them according to the priority you set. You may put one at a higher priority because it fits in with service development needs established in the business plan of the trust or practice, or put another lower because it does not fit in with other activities that your organisation has in their current development plan for the next 12 months. If you have identified a service development need by several different methods of assessment, or with several different patient groups or clinical conditions, then it will have a higher priority than something only identified once. Notify the service development needs you have identified to those responsible for agreeing and implementing the development plans of the trust and/or practice.

Look back at your aspirations and standards set out in Stages 1 and 2. Match your learning or service development needs with one or more of these standards, or others that you have set yourself.

## Stage 4: Make and carry out a learning and action plan with a timetable for your personal and service development

If you have not identified any learning needs for yourself or the service as a whole, you should omit Stage 4 and tidy up the presentation of your evidence for inclusion in your portfolio as at the end of Stage 5.

Think about whether:

- you have defined your learning objectives – what you need to learn to be able to attain the standards and outcomes you have described in Stage 2
- you can justify spending time and effort on the topics you prioritised in Stage 3. Is the topic important enough to your work, the NHS as a whole or patient safety? Does the clinical or non-clinical event occur sufficiently often to warrant the time spent?
- the time and resources for learning about that topic or making the associated changes to service delivery are available. Check that you are not trying to do too much too quickly, or you will become discouraged

- learning about that topic will make a difference to the care you or others can provide for patients
- how one topic fits in with other topics you have identified to learn more about. Have you achieved a good balance across your areas of work or between your personal aspirations and the basic requirements of the service?

Decide on what method of learning is most appropriate for your task or role or the standards you are expecting to attain or sustain. You may have already identified your preferred learning style – but read up on this if you are unsure.[10]

Describe how you will carry out your learning tasks and what you will do by a specified time. State how your learning will be applied and how and when it will be evaluated. Build in some staging posts so that you do not suddenly get to the end of 12 months and discover that you have only carried out half of your plan.

Your action plan should also include your role in remedying any gaps in service delivery that you identified in Stage 3 and that are within the remit of your responsibility.

## Stage 5: Document your learning, competence, performance and standards of service delivery

You might choose to document that you have attained your defined outcomes by repeating the learning needs assessment that you started with. You could record your increased confidence and competence in dealing with situations that you previously avoided or performed inadequately.

You might incorporate your assessment of what has been gained in a study of another area that overlaps.

# Preparing your portfolio

Use your professional portfolio to supply evidence of what you have learnt and to record standards of practice that:

- identify significant experiences that serve as important sources of learning
- reflect on the learning that arose from those experiences
- demonstrate learning in practice
- analyse and identify further learning needs and ways in which these needs can be met.

Your documentation might include all sorts of things, not just formal audits – although they make a good start. It might include reports of educational activities attended, statements of your roles and responsibilities, copies of publications you have read and critically appraised, and reports of your work. You could incorporate observations by others, evaluations of you observing other colleagues and how their practice differs from yours, descriptions of self-improvements, a video of typical activity, materials that demonstrate your skills to others, products of your input or learning – a new protocol for example. Box 1.4 gives a list of material you might include in your portfolio.

---

**Box 1.4:**   Possible contents of a portfolio
- Workload logs
- Case descriptions
- Videos
- Audiotapes
- Patient satisfaction surveys
- Research surveys
- Report of change or innovation
- Commentaries on published literature or books
- Records of critical incidents and learning points
- Notes from formal teaching sessions with reference to clinical work or other evidence

---

When you are preparing to submit your portfolio for a discussion with your manager (for example, at an appraisal) or for an assessment (for example, for a university post-registration award) write a self-assessment of your previous action plan. You might integrate your self-assessment into your PDP to show what you have achieved and what gaps you have still to address. Decide where are you now and where you want to be in one, three or five years.

Make sure all references are included and the documentation in your portfolio is as accurate and complete as possible. Organise how you have shown your learning steps and your standards of practice so that it is indexed and cross-referenced to the relevant sections of the paperwork. Discuss the contents of your portfolio with a colleague or a mentor to gain other people's perspectives of your work and look for blind spots.

## Reflective writing within the portfolio

Reflective writing has been endorsed by the NMC as an excellent way of analysing practice and learning from your everyday experiences.[2] Reflective writing can also be useful to analyse what you have learnt from attending formal learning sessions and considering how any newly acquired knowledge may be applied to practice. In order to provide a comprehensive structure to reflective writing, it is recommended that you adopt a model of reflection. This will help you to learn from your experience in a more logical and holistic manner. There are numerous models of reflection and it is best to choose a model that appears straightforward to you and seems to fit with your own style of thinking.[11-13]

Reflective writing introduces a personal element into your portfolio. It enables anyone reading the portfolio to gain insight into your practice. It is useful in creating a picture, which gives access to the artistry of nursing, and may demonstrate the therapeutic use of self in patient interactions.

## Include evidence of your competence as a practitioner with a special interest

You may have a particular expertise or special interest in a clinical field or non-clinical area such as management, teaching or research. It may be that you have a lead role or responsibility in your practice for chronic disease management of clinical conditions such as diabetes, asthma, mental health or coronary heart disease, or you may be employed by a PCO or hospital trust to:

- lead in the development of services
- deliver a procedure-based service
- deliver an opinion-based service.

The role of practitioner with special interest (PwSI) is being promoted by the Department of Health as a role that can help to bridge the gap between hospital and the community.[14] Realising the potential of nurses working in specialist roles will facilitate the redesign of primary care services. It may be particularly important for you, as a specialist, to be able to demonstrate your clinical expertise if you are seeking to gain a position as a PwSI. There is little consistency in the extent of training or qualifications at present within or across the various PwSI speciality areas.[14] Whatever your role, responsibility or expertise, your portfolio should include examples of evidence that show that you are competent, and that you have a consistently good performance in your speciality area. You may have parallel appraisals that you can include from your employer – for example, the university if you have a research or teaching post, or a hospital consultant if he or she supervises you in the clinical speciality.

When you gather evidence of your performance at work, try to document as many aspects of your work at one time as you can. When you are identifying what you need to learn, or gaps in service delivery, make sure that you involve patients and show how you interact with the team. This gives you evidence about 'relationships with patients' and 'working with colleagues' as well as the clinical area that you are focusing on or auditing.

# References

1  Nursing and Midwifery Council (2002) *Code of Professional Conduct*. Nursing and Midwifery Council, London.

2  Nursing and Midwifery Council (2001) *The PREP Handbook*. Nursing and Midwifery Council, London.

3  Wakley G, Chambers R and Field S (2000) *Continuing Professional Development in Primary Care*. Radcliffe Medical Press, Oxford.

4  Brown R (1995) *Portfolio Development and Profiling for Nurses* (2e). Quay Publishing, Wiltshire.

5  English National Board for Nursing, Midwifery and Health Visiting (1997) *Standards for Approval of Higher Education Institutions and Programmes*. English National Board for Nursing, Midwifery and Health Visiting, London.

6   Quinn F (2000) *Principles and Practice of Nurse Education* (4e). Stanley Thornes Ltd, London.

7   Nursing and Midwifery Council (2002) *Supporting Nurses and Midwives Through Lifelong Learning*. Nursing and Midwifery Council, London.

8   Royal College of General Practitioners/General Practitioners' Committee (2002) *Good Medical Practice for Practitioners*. Royal College of General Practitioners, London.

9   Nursing and Midwifery Council (1992) *Scope of Professional Practice*. Nursing and Midwifery Council, London.

10  Chambers R, Mohanna K, Wakley G and Wall D (2004) *Demonstrating Your Competence 1: healthcare teaching*. Radcliffe Medical Press, Oxford.

11  Gibbs G (1998) *Learning by Doing: a guide to teaching and learning methods*. Further Education Unit, Oxford Polytechnic, London.

12  Johns C (1996) Using a reflective model of nursing and guided reflection. *Nursing Standard*. **11(2)**: 34–8.

13  Schon D (1983) *The Reflective Practitioner: how professionals think in action*. Basic Books, New York.

14  Department of Health (2003) *Practitioners with Special Interests in Primary Care: implementing a scheme for nurses with special interests in primary care*. Department of Health, London. www.dh.gov.uk/assetRoot/04/07/23/69/04072369.pdf

# 2

## Practical ways to identify your learning and service needs as part of your portfolio

## Setting standards to show that you are competent

The Nursing and Midwifery Council (NMC) stresses the importance of lifelong learning. The council recognises that healthcare is an area of constant change which necessitates a dynamic approach to learning. In order to develop and maintain your competence you are required to 'demonstrate responsibility for your own learning through the development of a portfolio ... and to be able to recognise when further learning and development may be required'.[1]

You could make a good start by describing your current roles and responsibilities. This will help you to define what your competence should be now, or what competence you are hoping to attain (for instance as a specialist nurse). Once you have your definition, you can recognise whether you have, or lack in some part, the necessary competence. If there are no accepted descriptions of competence in the area you are focusing on, then you will have to start from scratch. You might compile your description using items from national guidelines such as in the National Service Frameworks or health strategies or the Agenda for Change.[2] The Department of Health has produced ideas relating to the role of nurses with special interests that you may find useful to adopt.[3]

Your definition of competence is likely to relate to your ability to undertake a task or role to a required standard. However, you will need to describe the standards expected in the range of tasks and roles you undertake and reference the source of standard setting. If professionals, or their organisations, are the only people involved in setting those standards, consider whether you should amend or extend the standards, tasks or roles by considering other perspectives, such as those of patients or your employing trust or practice.

There is a difference between being competent, and performing in a consistently competent manner. You need to be motivated to perform consistently well and enabled to do so with efficient systems and sufficient resources. You will require sufficient numbers of other competent healthcare professionals and available infrastructure such as diagnostic and treatment resources. It is partially your responsibility to alert managers to the resources needed to undertake your role effectively.

Choose methods in Stage 3 (*see* Chapter 1) to demonstrate your standards of performance and identify any learning needs that span different topic areas, to reduce duplication and maximise the usefulness of your learning. Collecting evidence of more than one aspect of your competence or performance cuts down the overall amount of work underpinning your PDP or included in your appraisal portfolio.

Use several methods to identify your learning needs and/or gaps in your service development or delivery, so that you validate the findings of one method by another. No one method will give you reliable information about the gaps in your knowledge, skills or attitudes or everyday service. Does what you think about your performance match with what others in the team or patients think of how you practise in your everyday work? It is particularly difficult to determine what it is you 'don't know you don't know' by yourself, yet it is vital that you identify and rectify those gaps. Other people may be able to tell you quite readily what you need to learn. Colleagues from different disciplines could usefully comment on any shortfalls in how your work interfaces with theirs.

Patients or people who don't use your services could tell you whether the way you work or provide services is off-putting or inappropriate. There may be data about your performance or your approach that could point out those gaps in your knowledge or skills of which you were previously unaware.

Determine what it is that you 'don't know you don't know' by:

- asking patients, users and non-users of your service
- comparing your performance against best practice or that of peers
- comparing your performance against objectives in business plans or national directives
- asking your peers, who perform a similar role, to observe and comment on your practice in a way that will identify both your strengths and weaknesses
- asking colleagues from different disciplines about shortfalls in how your work interfaces with theirs.

# Identify your learning needs – how you can find out if you need to be better at doing your job

You may decide to use a few selected methods to gather baseline evidence of your performance, focused on your specific area of expertise. Once you have identified your learning needs you will be able to create a flexible way to progress that takes account of your needs and circumstances. In order to establish your current position with a degree of objectivity you might use several of the methods described in this chapter such as:

- constructive feedback from peers or patients
- 360° feedback
- self-assessment, or review by others, using a rating scale to assess your skills and attitudes

- comparison with local or national protocols and guidelines for checking how well procedures are followed
- evaluative audit
- significant event audit
- eliciting patient views through methods such as satisfaction surveys
- a SWOT (strengths, weaknesses, opportunities and threats) or SCOT (strengths, challenges, opportunities and threats) analysis
- reading and reflecting
- educational review.

Several of these methods will also be useful for identifying any service development needs – you can look at the gaps identified from both the personal and service perspectives at the same time using the same method.

## Seek feedback

Find colleagues who will give you constructive feedback about your performance and practice. Don't be afraid to ask for comments on your style or work – just think how upsetting it would be if you were consistently doing something that irritated colleagues, but continued because nobody bothered to tell you the effect it was having. The golden rule for giving constructive feedback is to give positive praise of things that have been well done first. Sometimes colleagues launch straight in to criticise faults when asked for their views. The Pendleton model of giving feedback is widely used in the health setting (*see* Box 2.1):[4]

---

**Box 2.1:**   The Pendleton model of giving feedback[4]

1   The learner goes first and performs the activity.
2   The teacher questions or clarifies any facts.
3   The learner says what they thought was done well.
4   The teacher says what they thought was done well.
5   The learner says what could be improved upon.
6   The teacher says what could be improved upon.
7   Both discuss ideas for improvements in a helpful and constructive manner.

---

## 360° feedback

This collects together perceptions from a number of different participants as shown in Figure 2.1.

   The wider the spread of people giving feedback, the more rounded the picture. Each individual gives a feedback questionnaire to at least three people in each of the groups. An independent person then collects and collates the questionnaires and discusses the results with the individual. Computerised versions are available from commercial companies.[5] The main disadvantage of this method is that it can sometimes

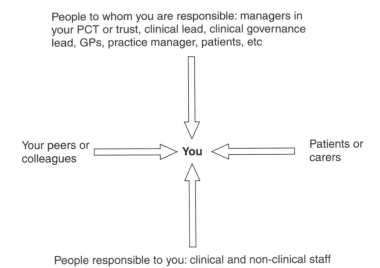

**Figure 2.1:**   360° feedback.

be spoilt by malicious comments against which individuals cannot readily defend themselves.

## Self-assess or gain another person's perspective on your standard of practice or service delivery

You might describe any aspect of your practice as statements (A to G as in Box 2.2) about your competence or performance, so that you can self-assess or others can give you feedback or comments by marking the extent to which they agree on the linear scales below. Objective feedback from external assessment is usually more reliable than your own self-assessment when you may have blind spots about your own performance. As you become more confident in this method of reviewing your competence, you might emphasise how consistent you are in your application of good practice – so in the statements below we have sometimes included 'consistently', 'always' or 'usually'. You can set your own challenges. If you have a mentor or a 'buddy' in the practice with whom you learn, you might discuss and reflect on the completed marking grids with him or her.

**Box 2.2:** Marking grid: circle the number which represents your views or feelings about each statement – complete the grid on more than one occasion and compare results over time

A  I consistently treat patients politely and with consideration.

STRONGLY AGREE                    to              STRONGLY DISAGREE

1------------------2------------------3------------------4------------------5------------------6

B  I am aware of how my personal beliefs could affect the care offered to the patient, and take care not to impose my own beliefs and values.

STRONGLY AGREE                    to              STRONGLY DISAGREE

1------------------2------------------3------------------4------------------5------------------6

C  I always treat all patients equally and ensure that some groups are not favoured at the expense of others.

STRONGLY AGREE                    to              STRONGLY DISAGREE

1------------------2------------------3------------------4------------------5------------------6

D  I try to maintain a relationship with the patient or family when a mistake has occurred.

STRONGLY AGREE                    to              STRONGLY DISAGREE

1------------------2------------------3------------------4------------------5------------------6

E  I always obtain informed consent to treatment.

STRONGLY AGREE                    to              STRONGLY DISAGREE

1------------------2------------------3------------------4------------------5------------------6

F  I usually involve patients in decisions about their care.

STRONGLY AGREE                    to              STRONGLY DISAGREE

1------------------2------------------3------------------4------------------5------------------6

G  I always respect the right of patients to refuse treatments or tests.

STRONGLY AGREE                    to              STRONGLY DISAGREE

1------------------2------------------3------------------4------------------5------------------6

## Compare your performance against protocols or guidelines

Are you familiar with all the protocols or guidelines that are used by someone, somewhere in your team? You might determine your learning needs and those of other team members by piling all the protocols or guidelines that exist in your team in a big heap and rationalising them so that you have a common set used by all. Working as a team you can compare your own knowledge and usual practice with others and with protocols or guidelines recommended by the National Institute for Clinical Excellence (NICE)[6] or National Service Frameworks or the Scottish Intercollegiate Guidelines Network (SIGN).[7]

Alternatively, you might compare your own practice against a protocol or guideline that is generally accepted at a national or local level. You could audit the standard of your practice to find out how often you adhere to such a protocol or guideline, and if you can justify why you deviate from the recommendations.

## Audit

Audit is:

> the method used by health professionals to assess, evaluate, and improve the care of patients in a systematic way, to enhance their health and quality of life.[8]

The five steps of the audit cycle are shown in Box 2.3.

---

**Box 2.3:**   The five steps of the audit cycle

1   Describe the criteria and standards you are trying to achieve.
2   Measure your current performance of how well you are providing care or services in an objective way.
3   Compare your performance against criteria and standards.
4   Identify the need for change – to performance, adjustment of criteria or standards, resources, available data.
5   Make any required changes as necessary and re-audit later.

---

Performance or practice is often broken down for the purposes of audit into the three aspects of structure, process and outcome. Structural audits might concern resources such as equipment, premises, skills, people, etc. Process audits focus on what is done to the patient: for instance, clinical protocols and guidelines. Audits of outcomes consider the impact of care or services on the patient and might include patient satisfaction, health gains and effectiveness of care or services. You might look at aspects of quality of the structure, process and outcome of the delivery of any clinical field, focusing on access, equity of care between different groups in the population, efficiency, economy, effectiveness for individual patients, etc.[8]

Set standards for your performance, find out how you are doing, search to find out best practice, make the changes and then re-audit the care given to patients in the future with the same problem. Some variations on audit include:

- *Case note analysis.* This gives an insight into your current practice. It might be a retrospective review of a random selection of notes, or a prospective survey of consecutive patients with the same condition as they present to see you.
- *Peer review.* Compare an area of your practice with other individual professionals or managers, or compare healthcare teams as a whole. An independent body might compare healthcare teams in one area e.g. within a primary care trust (PCT) or organisation so that like is compared with like. Feedback may be arranged to protect participants' identities so that only the individual person or team knows their own identity, the rest being anonymised, for example by giving each team a number. Where there is mutual trust and an open learning culture, peer review does not need to be anonymised and everyone can learn together about making improvements in practice.
- *Criteria-based audit.* This compares clinical practice with specific standards, guidelines or protocols. Re-audit of changes should demonstrate improvements in the quality of patient care.
- *External audit.* Prescribing advisers or managers in PCOs can supply information about indicators of performance for audit. Visits from external bodies such as the Healthcare Commission expose the PCO or hospital trust in England and Wales to external audit.
- *Tracer criteria.* Assessing the quality of care of a 'tracer' condition may be used to represent the quality of care of other similar conditions or more complex problems. Tracer criteria should be easily defined and measured. For instance, if you were to audit the extent to which you reviewed the treatment of menstrual bleeding problems, you might focus on a drug such as tranexamic acid and generalise from your audit results to your likely performance with other medications.

## Significant event audit

Think of an incident where a patient or you experienced an adverse event. This might be an unexpected death, an unplanned pregnancy, an avoidable side-effect from prescribed medication, a violent attack on a member of staff, or an angry outburst in public by you or a work colleague. You can review the case and reflect on the sequence of events that led to that critical event occurring. It is likely that there were a multitude of factors leading up to that significant event. You should take the case to a multidisciplinary meeting to reflect and analyse what were the triggers, causes and consequences of the event. Complete the significant event audit cycle by planning what individuals or the healthcare team as a whole might do to avoid a similar event happening in future. This might include undertaking further learning and/or making appropriate changes to your systems.

The steps of a significant event audit are shown in Box 2.4.

---

**Box 2.4:**   Steps of a significant event audit

- *Step 1*: Describe who was involved, what time of day, what the task/activity was, the context and any other relevant information.
- *Step 2*: Reflect on the effects of the event on the participants and the professionals involved.
- *Step 3*: Discuss the reasons for the event or situation arising with other colleagues, review case notes or other records.
- *Step 4*: Decide how you or others might have behaved differently. Describe your options for how the procedures at work might be changed to minimise or eliminate the event from recurring.
- *Step 5*: Plan changes that are needed, how they will be implemented, who will be responsible for what and when, what further training or resources are required. Then carry out the changes.
- *Step 6*: Re-audit later to see whether changes to procedures or new knowledge and skills are having the desired effects. Give feedback to the practice team.

---

## Assessment by an external body

This is a traditional way of showing that you are competent by taking and passing an examination. It is a good way of testing recalled knowledge in a written or oral examination, or establishing how you behave in a clinical situation on the day of a practical examination, but not much good for measuring anything else. A summative examination (i.e. done at the end of a course of study) gives a measure of your learning up to that date.

You might undertake an objective test of your knowledge and skills. Examples are a computer-based test in the form of multiple choice questions and patient management problems as in the nurse-prescribing website.[9] It may be worth considering subscribing to websites that provide multiple choice questionnaires that you can complete on paper and record this in your portfolio.[10]

## Elicit the views of patients

In striving to establish consistently good relationships with patients, you may assess patients' satisfaction with:

- you
- your practice
- the local hospital's way of working
- other services available in your locality.

Avoid surveys where questions are relatively superficial or biased. A more specific enquiry should uncover particular elements of patients' dissatisfaction, which will be more useful if you are trying to identify your learning needs. Use a well-validated patient questionnaire such as the General Practice Assessment Questionnaire (GPAQ) instead of risking producing your own version with ambiguities and flaws.[11] Many health professionals have used these patient survey methods, providing a bank of data against which to compare your performance.

Other sources of feedback from patients might be obtained through suggestion boxes for patients to contribute comments, or ask the team to record all patients' suggestions and complaints, however trivial, looking for patterns in the comments received.

There will be learning to be had from every complaint – even if the complaint does not have any substance, there should be something to learn about the shortfall in communication between you and the complainant.

The evolution of the 'expert patient programme' should mean that there is a pool of well-informed patients with chronic conditions who can contribute their insights into what you (or the service) need to learn from a patient's perspective.[12]

## Strengths, weaknesses (or challenges), opportunities and threats (SWOT or SCOT) analysis

You can undertake a SWOT (or SCOT) analysis of your own performance or that of your nursing team or healthcare organisation, working it out on your own, or with a workmate or mentor, or with a group of colleagues. Brainstorm the strengths, weaknesses (or challenges), opportunities and threats of your role or circumstances.

Strengths and weaknesses (or challenges) of your roles might relate to your clinical knowledge or skills, experience, expertise, decision making, communication skills, interprofessional relationships, political skills, timekeeping, organisational skills, teaching skills, or research skills. Strengths and weaknesses (or challenges) of the practice organisation might relate to most of these aspects as well as the way resources are allocated, overall efficiency and the degree to which the practice is patient centred.

Opportunities might relate to your unexploited experience or potential strengths, expected changes in the NHS, or resources for which you might bid. For example, you might train for and set up a special interest post.

Threats will include factors and circumstances that prevent you from achieving your aims for personal, professional and practice development or service improvements. They might be to do with your health, turnover in the team, or time-limited investment by your employing organisation.

List the important factors in your SWOT (or SCOT) analysis in order of priority through discussion with colleagues and independent people from outside your practice. Draw up goals and a timed action plan for you or the practice team to follow.

## Informal conversations – in the corridor, over coffee

You learn such a lot when chatting with colleagues at coffee time or over a meal, and can become aware of your learning or service development needs at these times. This is when you realise that other people are doing things differently from you and if they seem to be doing it better and achieving more, you can challenge yourself to decide if this matter could be one of your blind spots. Note down your thoughts before you forget them so that you can reflect on them later.

Online discussion groups may provide another source of informal exchanges with colleagues. If you find this difficult to start with, you might 'lurk', viewing the comments and views of other people until you feel confident enough to contribute. Record any observations that you find useful and reflect on how they might inform your own practice.

## Observe your work environment and role

Observation could be informal and opportunistic, or more systematic, working through a structured checklist. One method of self-assessment might be to audiotape yourself at work dealing with patients (after obtaining patients' informed consent). Listen to the tape afterwards to appraise your communication and consultation skills – on your own or with a friend or colleague. If you have access to video equipment, you might use this instead. You would need to discuss this in advance with your manager and comply with any policies on consent and confidentiality.

Look at the equipment that you use within your daily work. Do you know how to operate it properly? Assess yourself undertaking practical procedures, or ask someone to watch you operating the equipment or undertaking a practical procedure and give you feedback about your performance.

Analyse the various roles and responsibilities of your current posts. Compare your level of expertise against national standards such as in the Knowledge and Skills Framework or job evaluation framework as part of the Agenda for Change initiative.[13,14] Determine whether you can meet the requirements, or, if not, what deficiencies need to be made good.

You might combine one of the methods of identifying your learning needs already described such as an audit or SWOT analysis and apply it to 'observing your work environment or role', describing your relationship with other members of the multidisciplinary team for example, or reviewing how their roles and responsibilities interface with yours.

## Read and reflect

When reading articles in respected journals reflect on what the key messages mean for you in your situation. Note down topics about which you know little but that are relevant to your work, and calculate if you have further learning needs not met by the article you are reading. If the article is relevant to your practice, record what changes you will make and how you will make the changes. Record how you will impart your new knowledge to others in your team.

## Educational review

You might find a 'buddy' or work colleague, clinical tutor or someone who undertakes clinical supervision with you with whom you can have an informal or formal discussion about your performance, job situation and learning needs. You might draw up a learning contract as a result with a timed plan of action.

# Identify your service needs – how you can find out if there are gaps in services or how you deliver care

Now focus your attention on the needs of your practice or of your service organisation. The standards of service delivery should be those that allow you to practise as a competent clinician. You may be competent but be unable to perform or practise to a competent level if the resources available to you are inadequate, or other colleagues have insufficient knowledge or skills to support you. You cannot be expected to take responsibility for ensuring that resources you need to be able to practise in a competent manner are available. However, as a professional you should play a significant role in collecting evidence to make a case for the need for essential resources to your manager.

Some of the methods you might use are described below and include:

- involving patients and the public in giving you feedback about the quality and quantity of your services
- monitoring access and availability to care
- undertaking a force-field analysis
- assessing risk
- evaluating the standards of care or services you provide
- comparing the systems in your practice with those required by legislation
- considering your patient population's health needs
- reviewing teamwork
- assessing the quality of your services
- reflecting on whether you are providing cost-effective care and services.

## Involve patients and the public in giving you feedback about the quality and quantity of your services

Patient and public involvement may occur at three levels:

1  for individual patients about their own care
2  for patients and the public about the range and quality of health services on offer
3  in planning and organising health service developments.

The phrase 'patient and public involvement' is used here to mean individual involvement as a user, patient or carer, or public involvement that includes the processes of consultation and participation.[15]

If a patient involvement or public consultation exercise is to be meaningful, it has to involve people who represent the section of the population that the exercise is about. You will have to set up systems to actively seek out and involve people from minority groups or those with sensory impairments such as blind and deaf people.

Before you start:

- define the purpose

- be realistic about the magnitude of the planned exercise
- select an appropriate method or several methods depending on the target population and your resources
- obtain the commitment of everyone who will be affected by the exercise
- frame the method in accordance with your perspective
- write the protocol.

You might hold focus groups, or set up a patient panel, or invite feedback and help from a patient participation group. You could interview patients selected either at random from the patient population or for their experience of a particular condition or circumstance.

# Monitor access and availability to healthcare

## Access and availability

You could look at waiting times to see a health professional by using:

- computerised appointment lists or paper and pen to record the time of arrival, the time of the appointment, the time seen
- the next available appointments, which can easily be monitored by computer or, more painfully, by manual searches of the appointment books.

Compare the results at intervals (a spreadsheet is a good way to do this). Do you or other staff have learning needs in relation to the use of technology, or new ways of redesigning the service you offer?

## Referrals to other agencies and hospitals

You might audit and re-audit the time taken from the date the patient is seen to:

- the referral being sent (do you need more secretarial time?)
- the date the patient is seen by the other agency (could the patient be seen elsewhere quicker or do you need to liaise with other agencies over referrals?)
- the date the patient's needs have been met by investigation, diagnosis, treatment, provision of aid or support, etc (can you influence how quickly these are completed?).

Identify any learning needs here. For instance, new methods of teamwork with a different mix of skills between nurses, doctors and allied health professionals could provide extra services for your patients.

# Draw up a force-field analysis

This tool will help you to identify and focus down on the positive and negative forces in your work and to gain an overview of the weighting of these factors. Draw a horizontal or vertical line in the middle of a sheet of paper. Label one side 'positive' and the other side 'negative'. Draw bars to represent individual positive drivers that motivate you on one side of the line, and factors that are demotivating on the other negative side of the line. The thickness and length of the bars should represent the extent of the influence;

that is, a short, narrow bar will indicate that the positive or negative factor has a minor influence and a long, wide bar a major effect. *See* Box 2.5 for an example.

---

**Box 2.5:**   Example of force-field analysis diagram. Satisfaction with current post as a health professional

| Positive factors (driving forces) | Negative factors (restraining forces) |
|---|---|
| career aspirations | long hours of work |
| salary | demands from patients |
| autonomy | |
| satisfaction from caring | job insecurity |
| no uniform | oppressive hierarchy |
| opportunities for professional development | |

---

Take an overview of the resulting force-field diagram and consider if you are content with things as they are, or can think of ways to boost the positive side and minimise the negative factors. You can do this part of the exercise on your own, with a peer or a small group in the practice, or with a mentor or someone from outside the practice. The exercise should help you to realise the extent to which a known influence in your life, or in the practice as a whole, is a positive or negative factor. Make a personal or organisational action plan to create the situations and opportunities to boost the positive factors in your life and minimise the bars on the negative side.

## Assess risk

Risk assessment might entail evaluating the risks to the health or wellbeing or competence of yourself, staff and/or patients in your workplace, and deciding on the action needed to minimise or eliminate those risks.[16]

- *A hazard*: something with the potential to cause harm.
- *A risk*: the likelihood of that potential to cause harm being realised.

There are five steps to risk assessment:

1    look for and list the hazards
2    decide who might be harmed and how
3    evaluate the risks arising from the hazards and decide whether existing precautions are adequate or more should be done
4    record the findings
5    review your assessment from time to time and revise it if necessary.

You do not want to spend a lot of time and effort identifying risks or making changes if they do not matter much. When you have identified a risk, consider:

- is the risk large?
- does it happen often?
- is it a significant risk?

Risks may be prevented, avoided, minimised or managed where they cannot be eliminated. You, your colleagues and your staff may need to learn how to do this.

Record significant events where someone has experienced an adverse event or had a near miss – as part of you identifying your service development needs on an ongoing basis. Most significant incidents do not have one cause. Usually there are faults in the system, which are compounded by someone, or several people, being careless, tired, overworked or ill-informed. Cultivate an atmosphere of openness and discussion without blame, so that you can all learn from the significant event. If people think they will be blamed they will hide the incident and no one will be able to prevent it happening again. Look for *all* the causes and try to remedy as many as possible to prevent the situation from arising in the future.

## Evaluate the standards of services or care you provide

Keep your evaluation as simple as possible. Avoid wasting resources on unnecessarily bureaucratic evaluation. Design the evaluation so that you:

- specify the event (such as a service) to be evaluated – define broad issues, set priorities against strategic goals, time and resources, seek agreement on the nature and scope of the task
- describe the expected impact of the programme or activity and who will be affected
- define the criteria of success – these might relate to structure, process or outcome
- identify the information required to demonstrate the achievements of the programme or activity. The record might include: observing behaviour, data from existing records, prospective recording by the subjects of the programme or by the recipients and staff of the activity
- determine the time frame for the evaluation
- specify who collects the data for all stages in the delivery of the programme or activity, and the respective deadlines
- review and refine the objectives of the programme or activity and check that they are appropriate for the outcomes and impact you expect.

*What to evaluate?*

You could:

- Adopt any, or all, of the six aspects of the health service's performance assessment framework (*see* Box 2.6).
- Agree milestones and goals at stages in your programme or adopt others such as those relating to one of the National Service Frameworks.
- Evaluate the extent to which you achieve the outcome(s) starting with an objective. Alternatively, you might evaluate how conducive is the context of the programme, or activity, to achieving the anticipated outcomes.
- Undertake regular audits of aspects of the structure, process and outcome of a service or project to see if you have achieved what you expected when you established the criteria and standards of the audit programme.
- Evaluate the various components of a new system or programme: the activities, personnel involved, provision of services, organisational structure, precise goals and interventions.

---

**Box 2.6:** The six aspects of the NHS performance assessment framework

1   Health improvement
2   Fair access
3   Effective delivery
4   Efficiency
5   Patient/carer experience
6   Health outcomes

---

*Computer search*

The extent to which you can evaluate the practice of the healthcare team will depend on the quality of your records and the extent to which you use a computer to record healthcare information. In a general practice setting, for example, you could undertake a computerised search to identify those patients receiving oral contraceptives who have attended a contraceptive consultation within the practice over the past six months. In a hospital setting you could compare the duration of stay for patients undergoing particular surgery and analyse the reasons for variance. Make appropriate changes to your systems depending on what the computer search reveals. Put your plan into action and monitor with repeat searches at regular intervals.

Look at your learning or service development needs by analysing data from records to:

- look at trends and patterns of illness
- devise and use clinical guidelines and decision support systems as part of evidence-based practice
- audit what you are doing
- provide the information on which to base decisions on commissioning and management
- support epidemiology, research and teaching activities.

# Compare the systems in your workplace with those required by legislation

Legislation changes quite frequently. If you are employed within a large organisation such as an acute hospital, you can rely on managers to cascade information relating to legislative requirements down to you. In smaller organisations, such as general practice settings, you may need to raise awareness of legislative requirements. You could start by comparing the systems in your practice or workplace with those required by the Disability Discrimination Act[17] and health and safety legislation.[18]

# Consider your patients' health needs

Create a detailed profile of the local community that you serve. Ask your PCO or public health lead for information about practice populations and comparative information about the general population living in the district – morbidity and mortality statistics, referral patterns, age/sex mix, ethnicity, and population trends. You could also liaise with the wider community nursing service to investigate what information they hold relating to the health of the community.

Include information about the wider determinants of health such as housing, numbers of the population in, and types of, employment, geographical location, the environment, crime and safety, educational attainment and socio-economic data. Make a note of any particular health problems such as higher than average teenage pregnancy rates or drug misuse. If you work in a general practice setting, you could focus on the current state of health inequalities within your practice population or between your practice population and the district as a whole. It may be that circumstances change, which in turn alters the proportion of minority groups in a local area such as if a new adolescent care home opens up, or there is an influx of homeless people or asylum seekers into the locality.

# Review teamwork

You can measure how effective the team is – evaluate whether the team has:[19]

- clear goals and objectives
- accountability and authority
- individual roles for members
- shared tasks
- regular internal formal and informal communication
- full participation by members
- confrontation of conflict
- feedback to individuals
- feedback about team performance
- outside recognition
- two-way external communication
- team rewards.

## Assess the quality of your services

Quality may be subdivided into eight components: equity, access, acceptability and responsiveness, appropriateness, communication, continuity, effectiveness and efficiency.[20]

You might use the matrix in Box 2.7 as a way of ordering your approach to auditing a particular topic with the eight aspects of quality on the vertical axis and structure, process and outcome on the horizontal axis.[21] In this way you can generate up to 24 aspects of a particular topic. You might then focus on several aspects to look at the quality of patient care or services from various angles.

---

**Box 2.7:**    Matrix for assessing the quality of a clinical service

You might look at the structure, process or outcome of communicating test results to patients for example.

|  | Structure | Process | Outcome |
|---|---|---|---|
| Equity |  |  |  |
| Access |  |  |  |
| Acceptability and responsiveness |  |  |  |
| Appropriateness |  |  |  |
| Communication | Hospital report | Feedback | Action taken |
| Continuity |  |  |  |
| Effectiveness |  |  |  |
| Efficiency |  |  |  |

---

Look for service development needs reflecting why patients receive a poor quality of service such as:

- inadequately trained staff or staff with poor levels of competence
- lack of confidentiality
- staff not being trained in the management of emergency situations
- doctors or nurses not being contactable in an emergency or being ineffective
- treatment being unavailable due to poor management of resources or services
- poor management of the arrangements for home visiting
- insufficient numbers of available staff for the workload
- qualifications of locums or bank staff being unknown or inadequate for the posts they are filling
- arrangements for transfer of information from one team member to another being inadequate
- team members not acting on information received.

Many of these items will need action as a team, but for some of them it may be your responsibility to ensure that adequate standards are met.

# Reflect on whether you are providing cost-effective care and services

Cost-effectiveness is not synonymous with 'cheap'. A cost-effective intervention is one that gives a better or equivalent benefit from the intervention in question for lower or equivalent cost, or where the relative improvement in outcome is higher than the relative difference in cost. In other words being cost-effective means having the best outcomes for the least input. Using the term 'cost-effective' implies that you have considered potential alternatives.

An intervention must first be considered *clinically* effective to warrant investigation into its potential to be *cost*-effective. Evidence-based practice must incorporate clinical judgement. You have to interpret the evidence when it comes to applying it to individual patients, whether it is evidence about clinical effectiveness or cost-effectiveness. A new or alternative treatment or intervention should be compared directly with the previous best treatment or intervention.

An economic evaluation is a comparative analysis of two or more alternatives in terms of their costs and consequences. There are four different types as shown in Box 2.8.

---

**Box 2.8:**    The four types of economic evaluation

1   *Cost-effectiveness analysis* is used to compare the effectiveness of two interventions with the same treatment objectives.
2   *Cost minimisation* compares the costs of alternative treatments that have identical health outcomes.
3   *Cost–utility analysis* enables the effects of alternative interventions to be measured against a combination of life expectancy and quality of life; common outcome measures are quality adjusted life years (QALYs) or health-related quality of life (hrqol).
4   *Cost–benefit analysis* is a technique designed to determine the feasibility of a project, plan, management or treatment by quantifying its costs and benefits. It is often difficult to determine these accurately in relation to health.

---

While health valuation is unavoidable, it cannot be objective. You will probably have learning needs around what subjective method is best to use.[22]

Efficiency is sometimes confused with effectiveness. Being efficient means obtaining the most quality from the least expenditure, or the required level of quality for the least expenditure. To measure efficiency you need to make a judgement about the level of quality of the 'purchase' and be able to relate it to 'price'. 'Price' alone does not measure efficiency. Quality is the indicator used in combination with price to assess if something is more efficient. So, cost-effectiveness is a measure of efficiency and suggests that costs have been related to effectiveness.

Consider if you have service development needs. Discuss whether:

*   the current skill mix in your team is appropriate

- more cost-effective alternative types of delivery of care are available
- sufficient staff training exists for those taking on new roles and responsibilities.

# Set priorities: how you match what's needed with what's possible

You and your colleagues will have been able to make a wish list after following the previous Stages 3A and 3B undertaking a variety of needs assessments. Group and summarise your learning and service development needs from the exercises you have carried out. Grade them according to the priority you set. You may put one at a higher priority because it fits in with learning needs established from another section, or put another lower because it does not fit in with other activities that you will put into your learning plan for the next 12 months. If you have identified a learning need by several different methods of assessment then it will have a higher priority than something only identified once in your PDP. Collect information from all the team, the patients, users and carers, to feed back before you make a decision on how to progress. Remember to take external influences into account, such as the National Service Frameworks, NICE guidance, governmental priorities, priorities of your PCO, the content of the Local Delivery Plan, etc.

Select those topics that are tied into organisational priorities, have clear aims and objectives and are achievable within your time and resource constraints. When ranking topics for learning or action in order of priority (Stage 4) consider whether:

- the project aims and objectives are clearly defined
- the topic is important:
  - for the population served (e.g. the size of the problem and/or its severity)
  - for the skills, knowledge or attitudes of the individual or team
- it is feasible
- it is affordable
- it will make enough difference
- it fits in with other priorities.

You will still have more ideas than can possibly be implemented. Remember the highest priority – the health service is for patients that use it or who will do so in the future.

# References

1   Nursing and Midwifery Council (2002) *Supporting Nurses and Midwives Through Lifelong Learning.* Nursing and Midwifery Council, London.

2   www.rcn.org.uk/agendaforchange

3   Department of Health (2003) *Practitioners with Special Interests.* Department of Health, London.

4   Pendleton D, Schofield T, Tate P and Havelock P (2003) *The New Consultation: developing doctor–patient communication.* Oxford University Press, Oxford.

5  King J (2002) Career focus: 360° appraisal. *British Medical Journal.* **324**: S195.

6  National Institute for Clinical Excellence (NICE) www.nice.org.uk

7  Scottish Intercollegiate Guidelines Network (SIGN) www.sign.ac.uk

8  Irvine D and Irvine S (eds) (1991) *Making Sense of Audit.* Radcliffe Medical Press, Oxford.

9  www.nurse-prescriber.co.uk/mcq.htm

10  www.eguidelines.co.uk

11  www.npcrdc.man.ac.uk

12  Department of Health (2003) *EPP Update Newsletter.* Department of Health, London. See Expert Patient Programme on www.ohn.gov.uk/ohn/people/expert.htm

13  Department of Health (2003) *The NHS Knowledge and Skills Framework (NHS KSF) and Development Review Guidance – working draft* Version 6. Department of Health, London.

14  Department of Health (2003) *Job Evaluation Handbook* Version 1. Department of Health, London.

15  Chambers R, Drinkwater C and Boath E (2002) *Involving Patients and the Public: how to do it better* (2e). Radcliffe Medical Press, Oxford.

16  Mohanna K and Chambers R (2000) *Risk Matters in Healthcare.* Radcliffe Medical Press, Oxford.

17  Her Majesty's Government (1995) Disability and Discrimination Act. The Stationery Office, London. www.hmso.gov.uk/acts/acts1995/1995050.htm

18  www.hse.gov.uk

19  Hart E and Fletcher J (1999) Learning how to change: a selective analysis of literature and experience of how teams learn and organisations change. *Journal of Interprofessional Care.* **13(1)**: 53–63.

20  Maxwell RJ (1984) Quality assessment in health. *British Medical Journal.* **288**: 1470–2.

21  Firth-Cozens J (1993) *Audit in Mental Health Services.* LEA, Howe.

22  McCulloch D (2003) *Valuing Health in Practice.* Ashgate Publishing Ltd, Aldershot.

# 3

## Demonstrating common components of good quality healthcare

In looking at the quality of care you provide and demonstrating your standards of service delivery and outcomes of learning, you should find that obtaining informed consent from patients for their treatment, maintaining confidentiality and handling complaints are part of the fabric of good quality care. We have considered them separately in this chapter, but each may be individualised to any of the seven clinical areas of Chapters 4 to 10.

We have set out the chapter with key information about consent followed by some example cycles of the stages of evidence (*see* Figure 1.1 on page 6). The two other sections on confidentiality and complaints follow, laid out in similar ways. Read through the cycles of evidence to become familiar with the approach to gathering and documenting evidence of your learning, competence, performance or standards of service delivery. Then either adopt one of the examples or adapt it to your own circumstances. Alternatively, read on to one or more of the clinical chapters and look at these three components in a clinical context such as in relation to contraception or sexually transmitted infections in Chapters 5 and 6.

# Consent

## Key points

Information given to a health professional remains the property of the patient. In most circumstances, consent is assumed for the necessary sharing of information with other professionals involved with the care of the patient for that episode of care. Usually consent is also assumed for essential sharing of information for continuing care. Beyond this, informed consent must be obtained. Patients attend for healthcare in the belief that the personal information that they supply, or which is found out about them during investigation or treatment, will be confidential. The NMC *Code of Professional Conduct* provides specific advice on protecting confidential information.[1]

Confidential information may be disclosed in the following circumstances:[1]

- if the patient consents
- if it is in the patient's own interest that information should be disclosed, but it is either impossible to seek the patient's consent or

- it is medically undesirable in the patient's own interest, to seek the patient's consent
- if the law requires (and does not merely permit) the health professional to disclose the information
- if disclosure is needed for the interest of the public (e.g. in order to protect the patient from risk of harm)
- in issues of child protection, in which case you must act within local and national policies.

> Health professionals must be able to justify their decision to disclose information without consent. If they are in any doubt, they should consult their professional bodies and colleagues.

Consent is only valid if the patient fully understands the nature and consequences of disclosure – they must be able to give their consent, receive enough information to enable them to make a decision and be acting under their own free will and not persuaded by the strong influence of another person. If consent is given, the health worker is responsible for limiting the disclosure to that information for which informed consent has been obtained. The development of modern information technology and the increasing amount of multidisciplinary teamwork in patient care make confidentiality difficult to uphold.

You may need to give information about a patient to a relative or carer. Normally the consent of the patient should be obtained. Sometimes, the clinical condition of the patient may prevent informed consent being obtained (e.g. they are unconscious or have a severe illness). It is important to recognise that relatives or carers do *not* have any right to information about the patient. Disclosure without consent may be justified when third parties are exposed to a risk so serious that it outweighs the patient's privacy. An example would be if a patient declines to allow you to disclose information about their health and continues to drive against medical advice when unfit to do so.

Local research ethics committees and the research governance framework ensure best practice in the giving of informed consent by patients in research studies.

As health professionals, we often assume implied consent. The general public and patients are generally ignorant of the extent to which information about them is passed around the NHS. When teaching at both pre-registration and post-registration levels, in examinations and assessments and in research we may incorrectly assume patients imply their consent. Consent is also implied for health service accounting, central monitoring of referrals, in disease registers, for audit and in facilitating joint working between team members. The NHS is still engaged in a debate about what data can legitimately be shared without patients' explicit consent. Although written consent is usually obtained for supplying information to insurance companies or for legal reports, patients are often unaware of the type of information being supplied and may not have not given 'informed consent'.

Consent to treatment with medication is also often assumed – the doctor or nurse prescribes the medication and the patient takes it.[2] However, we know that a prescription may not be taken to the pharmacy for dispensing, or if it is, the medication is not started, or continued. You need to think about how you move from compliance to concordance as defined below:

- *compliance* with treatment or lifestyle changes implies that the patient follows instructions from health professionals to a greater or lesser degree
- *concordance* is a negotiated agreement on treatment between the patient and the healthcare professional. It allows patients to take informed decisions on the degree of risk or suffering that they themselves wish to undertake or follow.

Seeking consent is a fundamental part of good practice, and issues around validity and capacity to consent are covered in greater depth in the Department of Health reference guide or can be explored on their website.[3]

# Collecting data to demonstrate your learning, competence, performance and standards of service delivery: consent

## Example cycle of evidence 3.1

- Focus: informed consent
- Other relevant focus: relationships with patients

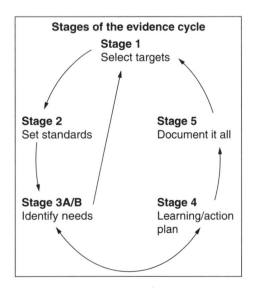

**Stages of the evidence cycle**

**Stage 1**
Select targets

**Stage 2**
Set standards

**Stage 3A/B**
Identify needs

**Stage 4**
Learning/action plan

**Stage 5**
Document it all

---

**Case study 3.1**

Mrs Bowed comes to see the practice nurse about her contraception. The nurse sketches out the alternatives that are open to her as a 35-year-old smoker. It transpires that she has had unprotected sexual intercourse four days previously and is at risk of pregnancy. The nurse advises having an intrauterine device (IUD) fitted straightaway, as this will provide emergency contraception and long-term contraception. 'You might as well – you know best,' says Mrs Bowed passively, with a long sigh. Further discussion reveals that Mrs Bowed felt pressured to have a termination of pregnancy by her mother when a teenager, with which the doctors colluded. Since then, she's never taken any real decisions about her health or contraception, having had a domineering husband who has recently left her.

---

This is just an example. Keep your task simple. You could choose three or four cycles of evidence to demonstrate your competence each year.

*Stage 1: Select your aspirations for good practice*

The excellent nurse:

* obtains informed consent before treatment
* treats patients politely and with consideration.

*Stage 2: Set the standards for your outcomes*

---

Outcomes might include:

* the way learning is applied
* a learnt skill
* a protocol
* a strategy that is implemented
* meeting recommended standards.

---

* A completed audit that shows that you, or all clinicians in the team, consistently obtain women's informed consent to treatment or other clinical management.

- Devise, apply and act on appropriate patient surveys that ascertain patients' views about their treatment by health professionals e.g. establishing views as to whether you treat patients politely and with consideration.
- You might choose to focus on consent for contraception such as an injection, the fitting of an IUD or implant, or for investigations such as taking vaginal swabs.

## Stage 3A: Identify your learning needs

- Review the consent and communication issues in a complaint or expression of discontent made by a patient to any member of the practice team.
- Reflect on whether you follow best practice in obtaining and recording consent to treatment or procedures.

## Stage 3B: Identify your service needs

Any of the needs assessment exercises in 3A may also reveal service needs.

- Compare the consent policy in your particular area of practice against best practice recommendations from the NMC,[1] and consent policies from other NHS trusts, and reflect on the differences.
- Audit the case notes to determine whether doctors and nurses recorded the discussion of parental knowledge and consent to treatment with contraception in consultations with under-16 year olds in line with the Fraser guidelines.[4]
- Undertake a targeted teenage patient survey. You might look at teenagers who have consulted general practitioners (GPs) or nurses at a local surgery or family planning clinic. Alternatively, you might learn more from a survey of teenagers at a local youth centre, as this would include non-users of GP services. You could ask about any aspect of teenage health, such as their experiences of informed consent, or how treatment options have been explained, or their experience of consultations with local GPs or nurses, relating to politeness and consideration.

## Stage 4: Make and carry out a learning and action plan

- Identify the issues from the learning and service needs assessment exercises in Stages 3A and 3B, e.g. comparing your own consent policy with others.
- Set up a workshop on communication skills highlighting politeness and consideration, and ability to gain informed consent, e.g. by video recording and reflection/feedback with various types of patients including teenagers (with their informed consent!).
- Arrange and attend a facilitated meeting with a group of women to discuss their experiences of consulting health professionals, to gain their opinions about access, the welcome, and general attitudes e.g. organised by the practice's patient participation group.

*Stage 5: Document your learning, competence, performance and standards of service delivery*

• Make notes of the review of the complaint or adverse comments and subsequent plan to minimise likelihood of re-occurrence.
• Repeat the initial learning or service needs assessments, e.g. re-audit and repeat the patient survey.
• Audit that the consent policy is applied consistently by all clinical members of the practice team, e.g. from case notes, patient feedback, self-report. You might find that consent is reported as being obtained but not recorded in the patients' records. This would imply that a change in recording practice is required and produce future new learning needs!

---

**Case study 3.1 continued**

You help Mrs Bowed to understand the risk and consequences of pregnancy and the urgency of action she needs to take if she wishes to receive emergency contraception. You talk through the advantages and disadvantages of the fitting of an IUD and its use as long-term contraception. You suggest an assertiveness course she might like to consider, run by the local further education college. You arrange for the IUD to be fitted later the same day when she has had an opportunity to reflect about what she wants to do and has given informed consent to the fitting.

---

# Example cycle of evidence 3.2

• Focus: informed consent
• Other relevant focus: research

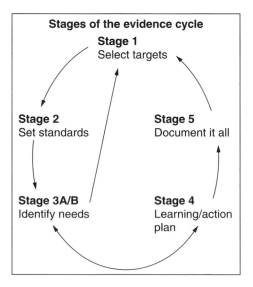

**Stages of the evidence cycle**

**Stage 1**
Select targets

**Stage 2**
Set standards

**Stage 3A/B**
Identify needs

**Stage 4**
Learning/action plan

**Stage 5**
Document it all

> **Case study 3.2**
>
> The practice team with whom you work decides to undertake a survey to find out if patients are satisfied with the service they receive. The practice manager will organise it, but you are nominated to lead the work. You decide to focus on teenagers as a group as the adolescent drop-in clinic you set up two years ago with the school health service is not being used as much as it once was. You are not sure how to survey the teenagers. You think they are unlikely to answer questionnaires sent through the post and think you will interview teenagers about their satisfaction with the clinic. You intend to employ one of your own teenage children to interview some who have never come to the clinic by selecting their names from your patient list as well as some teenagers who have attended. You're not sure if you are getting into research territory or if it is okay to claim you are auditing your services.

This is just an example. Keep your task simple. You could choose three or four cycles of evidence to demonstrate your competence each year.

## Stage 1: Select your aspirations for good practice

The excellent nurse:

- protects patients' rights and makes sure that they are not disadvantaged by taking part in research
- gives patients the information they need about their problem in a way they can understand as a basis for informed consent.

## Stage 2: Set the standards for your outcomes

Outcomes might include:

- the way learning is applied
- a learnt skill
- a protocol
- a strategy that is implemented
- meeting recommended standards.

- A practice policy of informed consent covers patients' participation in audit and research as well as consent to clinical treatment.

- You are able to describe the difference between audit of clinical management and service provision and research.

## Stage 3A: Identify your learning needs

- Read through the frequently asked questions and answers on the Department of Health website relating to research governance.[5] Consider whether you are able to answer the questions before reading the answers.
- Describe an audit plan of an adolescent clinic that involves obtaining young people's views of standards of services by interviewing them. Submit the plan to the chair of the local research ethics committee to check that he/she agrees that the audit proposal does not fall within the definition of research and to approve the patient literature and the process inviting informed consent to take part.

## Stage 3B: Identify your service needs

Any of the needs assessment exercises in 3A may also reveal service needs.

- Draw up an information leaflet for young people about the audit of adolescent clinic services that you intend to carry out. Ask others to critique the leaflet – young people for its readability and clarity, a research colleague for the extent to which it conforms to best practice for informed consent. Use the information leaflet so that they can give informed consent to the interview to obtain their views and audio recording of the interview.
- Ask a colleague to peer review the extent to which advice and information you give to teenagers during a consultation is accurate. The teenager would need to have given prior, written informed consent for the peer review (and audio recording if used).

## Stage 4: Make and carry out a learning and action plan

- Obtain and read documents about research governance from the Department of Health's website or from your PCO – as in section 3A (first part).
- Study the application form for the ethical approval of a research study.
- Understand the limits to obtaining patients' views as part of audit of clinical and service management by reading up on informed consent. Look at whether you are routinely explaining the details of a diagnosis or prognosis, and consider whether you routinely liaise with medical colleagues to discover what information they have given to patients. Consider whether you always give an explanation of likely benefits and side-effects of treatment, and what will happen if no treatment is given. Ensure that patients are always made to understand if a proposed treatment is experimental and if students in training will be involved in their care.
- Arrange to meet with your local clinical governance lead and ask about good practice in obtaining patients' views through audit, research and patient involvement activities – including good practice in informed consent.

*Stage 5: Document your learning, competence, performance and standards of service delivery*

- Make a comparison of your own practice with the answers to the frequently asked questions on the Department of Health website relating to research governance.[5]
- File the response letter from the chair of the local research ethics committee about the audit proposal.
- Keep the subsequent revised audit plan to ensure that work does not fall within the definition of research.
- Keep the revised patient's informed consent leaflet, following the critique.
- Repeat the peer review by the same or another colleague, of the extent to which advice and information you give to teenagers during consultations is accurate.

---

**Case study 3.2 continued**

The chair of the research ethics committee advises you that your plan should be classed as research rather than audit as it involves contact with patients outside their usual NHS care. He explains about the risks of using untrained interviewers such as your own children and the need to fully inform those teenagers you are inviting to be interviewed about the survey, and that their refusal will not prejudice their medical care. He advises you to send an application form for formal approval to the ethics committee and to contact the research lead in your PCO in line with the research governance framework if you wish to continue to develop a research project. You revise your plans as the scale of the work required is becoming out of all proportion.

---

# Example cycle of evidence 3.3

- Focus: communication skills
- Other relevant foci: informed consent, working with colleagues

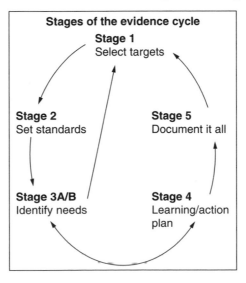

**Stages of the evidence cycle**

**Stage 1**
Select targets

**Stage 2**
Set standards

**Stage 5**
Document it all

**Stage 3A/B**
Identify needs

**Stage 4**
Learning/action plan

> **Case study 3.3**
>
> Miss Young, who has severe learning difficulties, comes with her carer to have a cervical smear undertaken. The carer explains that the surgery has written to Miss Young stating that she is overdue for a smear. Looking at Miss Young's medical records, you discover that she has never had a smear although she is now 52 years old. You wonder how to proceed, as Miss Young's carer tells you that Miss Young has been sexually active for some time. The carer seems to be convinced that it will be in Miss Young's best interests for her have the smear test undertaken but Miss Young herself does not seem to be aware of why smear tests are important.

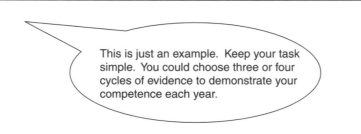

This is just an example. Keep your task simple. You could choose three or four cycles of evidence to demonstrate your competence each year.

## Stage 1: Select your aspirations for good practice

The excellent nurse:

- acts in the best interests of patients when providing or arranging treatment or care, acting with patients' informed consent
- makes sure that others understand their professional status and speciality, what roles and responsibilities they have and who is responsible for each aspect of the patient's care
- acts as the patient's advocate
- clarifies the criteria for taking cervical smears.

## Stage 2: Set the standards for your outcomes

> Outcomes might include:
>
> - the way learning is applied
> - a learnt skill
> - a protocol
> - a strategy that is implemented
> - meeting recommended standards.

- Obtain acceptance of a policy from the practice team on informed consent for patients with mental health problems and learning disabilities.

## Stage 3A: Identify your learning needs

- Analyse a significant event, e.g. you established that Miss Young is at risk of developing cervical cancer. You agree to undertake the screening procedure as Miss Young's carer tells you that Miss Young has given consent for the procedure. However, when you attempt to take the smear Miss Young becomes unco-operative. One of Miss Young's relatives later complains that you tried to force her to have a cervical smear to keep your numbers up.
- Self-assessment – you are aware that you do not know how to proceed (e.g. in the consultation in the case study). You do not know how much you can rely on the carer telling you that Miss Young has given informed consent or the extent to which you can take Miss Young's initial acquiescence for 'consent'.
- Read up and reflect on the association between competency or capacity to be well informed and the degree of previous education and the inability of some individuals to provide informed consent if they have educational, social and cultural reasons that limit their understanding of complex issues.

## Stage 3B: Identify your service needs

> Any of the needs assessment exercises in 3A may also reveal service needs.

- Carry out a review of case notes of women aged 20–65 years with learning disabilities, to determine the numbers who have had cervical smears, mammograms, immunisations, etc.
- Arrange a focus group discussion with other health professionals, people with learning disabilities and their carers (or other target group such as people with dementia and their carers), to discuss the appropriateness of the patient's consent process for all clinical interventions including cervical cytology and mammography.

## Stage 4: Make and carry out a learning and action plan

- Ask advice from MENCAP about the approach they recommend for obtaining informed consent from 'vulnerable' groups of people, how to explain clinical management and pursue clinical interventions, together with any associated useful literature.[6]
- Read up on informed consent.
- Revise the practice informed consent policy to include specific groups of 'vulnerable' people such as those with learning disabilities or mental ill-health problems.

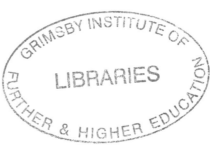

*Stage 5: Document your learning, competence, performance and standards of service delivery*

- Run a quiz for members of the practice team at an in-house educational event with four hypothetical cases. Compare the answers with best practice according to MENCAP and other professional literature.[6]
- Include the revised practice policy on informed consent.
- Audit the consistent application of the revised practice informed consent policy with consecutive cases, e.g. search on people coded as having learning disability on computer. Look to see what interventions have been undertaken and whether informed consent has been recorded in the notes.
- Include in your portfolio specimen consent forms that have been piloted, revised and audited.

---

**Case study 3.3 continued**

Miss Young returns for a follow-up appointment, having left after the previous surgery appointment to think about having a cervical smear. She has told her carer that she has had some bleeding from down below so a pelvic examination and smear are warranted clinically. You take plenty of time to explain how you will do the pelvic examination and smear, Miss Young agrees and all goes well.

---

# Confidentiality

## Key points

You should have appropriate confidentiality safeguards in place in the practice to prevent inadvertent disclosure of personal and sensitive information about patients. Tell people, especially the young, about their right to confidential medical treatment and reinforce your conversation with posters and leaflets. People with non-prescription drug-related problems who seek help from substance abuse clinics, or those with sexually transmitted infections who attend genitourinary medicine clinics, often do not want their GP to be told because they do not believe that the information will be kept confidential. Fears about confidentiality are the commonest reason young people give for not attending their general practice surgery for contraceptive treatment.[7]

Young people under the age of 16 years have the same rights to confidentiality as other patients. The younger the person, the greater care that is needed to assess the level of understanding to ensure that he or she understands the consequences of any proposed action. If a young person fulfils the conditions given in Box 3.1 he or she is regarded as being competent to make his or her own decisions.

---

**Box 3.1:** The Fraser guidelines[4]

The guidelines were drawn up after Lord Fraser stated in 1985 that a health professional could give contraceptive advice or treatment to a person under 16 years old without parental consent, providing that the professional is satisfied that:

- the young person will understand the advice
- the young person cannot be persuaded to tell their parents or allow the doctor to tell them that they are seeking contraceptive advice
- the young person is likely to begin or continue having unprotected sex with or without contraceptive treatment
- the young person's physical or mental health is likely to suffer unless they receive contraceptive advice or treatment
- it is in the young person's best interest to receive contraceptive advice or treatment.

The Fraser guidelines apply to health professionals in England and Wales. In Scotland, the Age of Legal Capacity (Scotland) Act 1991 gives similar powers of consent to those under 16 years of age.

In Northern Ireland, although separate legislation applies, the then Department of Health and Social Services Northern Ireland stated that there was no reason to suppose that the Northern Ireland Courts would not follow the House of Lords' decision.

---

Occasionally you may feel that you have a moral obligation to divulge confidential information. Whenever possible you should seek to persuade the patient to give consent to the disclosure. Seek advice from your professional organisations in circumstances where others are at danger (e.g. risk of harm, or rape or sexual abuse), or where a serious crime has been committed. Health professionals should satisfy themselves that sufficient authority has been obtained (e.g. a certificate from the Attorney General or Lord Advocate) and consult colleagues and professional organisations before disclosing information without a patient's consent.

The Caldicott Committee Report described principles of good practice to safeguard confidentiality when information is being used for non-clinical purposes:[8]

- justify the purpose
- do not use patient-identifiable information unless it is absolutely necessary
- use the minimum necessary patient-identifiable information
- access to patient-identifiable information should be on a strict need-to-know basis
- everyone with access to patient-identifiable information should be aware of his or her responsibilities.

Interpreters should be used wherever possible to avoid the use of friends or relatives. They should be trained in the requirements of confidentiality.

Patients are entitled to access data held about them. Exceptions to this right are:

- the patient failed to make the request in accordance with the Data Protection Act 1998
- if acceding to the request would result in disclosure of information about somebody else without their consent
- when giving medical information may cause serious harm to the mental or physical health of the patient (a rare occurrence).

You need to incorporate systems for ensuring that paper and computer security are maintained. Systems for monitoring and upgrading security systems should be in place and you should check regularly that confidentiality is not being breached if changes are made.

# Collecting data to demonstrate your learning, competence, performance and standards of service delivery: confidentiality

## Example cycle of evidence 3.4

- Focus: confidentiality
- Other relevant focus: teaching and training

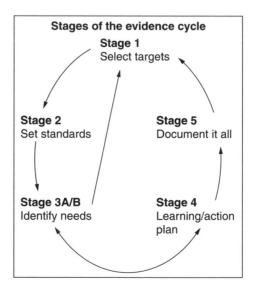

> **Case study 3.4**
>
> It is the first time you have had student nurses placed with you and you want to ensure that they are aware of the professional guidelines on confidentiality, and teach them about the importance of making sure that young people understand the practice code on confidentiality while they are on their placement with you.

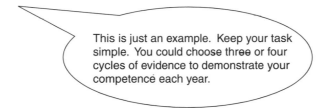

This is just an example. Keep your task simple. You could choose three or four cycles of evidence to demonstrate your competence each year.

## Stage 1: Select your aspirations for good practice

The excellent nurse:
- maintains the confidentiality of patient-specific information
- ensures that patients are aware of when they are receiving care from students and are not put at risk.

## Stage 2: Set the standards for your outcomes

Outcomes might include:

- the way learning is applied
- a learnt skill
- a protocol
- a strategy that is implemented
- meeting recommended standards.

- Ensure that all members of the practice team including you, new members of staff and students or doctors in training are familiar with guidelines for confidentiality in relation to patients receiving healthcare.

## Stage 3A: Identify your learning needs

- Assess your knowledge about the limits of confidentiality, e.g. for providing under-16 year olds with contraception or referring them for termination of pregnancy or other surgical interventions.

- Ask a colleague who has teaching experience how you could best approach an in-house training session on maintaining confidentiality for teenagers of different ages, which will convey the most important messages and lead to changes where necessary.

## Stage 3B: Identify your service needs

Any of the needs assessment exercises in 3A may also reveal service needs.

- Compare the practice protocol for confidentiality with the guidelines in the *Confidentiality and Young People* toolkit.[7]
- Review the intended induction programme for new members of staff, including administrative staff, students on placement and doctors in training, to assess the extent to which knowledge of confidentiality features and is addressed.

## Stage 4: Make and carry out a learning and action plan

- Talk to community practice educators about how to undertake learning needs assessments of others from different disciplines with different levels of responsibilities in respect of confidentiality.
- Prepare for and run an interactive teaching session on confidentiality for patients of all age groups with special focus on teenagers. You might invite the whole practice team, including students, family planning or school nurses, local pharmacists, GP registrars, etc. You could use the *Confidentiality and Young People* toolkit for promoting discussion with the practice team at the session. You could use a quiz before and after the session to evaluate the effectiveness of the session.[7]

## Stage 5: Document your learning, competence, performance and standards of service delivery

- Include the results from the quiz completed by those attending the teaching session before and after training about confidentiality.
- Keep an incident record kept by the practice team of any reported or perceived breaches of confidentiality by anyone working in, or associated with, the practice.
- Record the existence of personal learning plans based on learning needs assessments for new staff or doctors in training by the end of their induction period.
- Include in your records the revised practice protocol in line with the *Confidentiality and Young People* toolkit.[7]

---

**Case study 3.4 continued**

Other staff colleagues join your teaching session with the students using the video from the *Confidentiality and Young People* toolkit.[7] All get full marks in the quiz after watching the video.

---

# Learning from complaints

## Key points

Even if a complaint is trivial or undeserved, it implies a lack of communication. The basis of any complaints procedure should be about good communication. There is learning to be had from every complaint. Complaints are often addressed defensively because of fear of criticism or litigation.[9] Poor communication is likely to generate misunderstandings and good communication can help to diffuse difficult situations. Often the complainant is merely looking for an opportunity to give full expression to his concerns and to establish an opportunity to gain the full facts. Many complaints highlight failings in systems and processes that can be easily altered to prevent repetition of error.

# Collecting data to demonstrate your learning, competence, performance and standards of service delivery: complaints

## Example cycle of evidence 3.5

- Focus: complaints
- Other relevant focus: working with colleagues

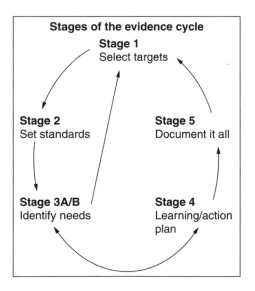

Stages of the evidence cycle

Stage 1
Select targets

Stage 2
Set standards

Stage 5
Document it all

Stage 3A/B
Identify needs

Stage 4
Learning/action plan

---

**Case study 3.5**

The clinic where you work has received a patient complaint about lack of privacy for patients when having cervical smears taken by a locum nurse. This has prompted you all as a practice team to review the way that your complaints system functions.

---

This is just an example. Keep your task simple. You could choose three or four cycles of evidence to demonstrate your competence each year.

## *Stage 1: Select your aspirations for good practice*

The excellent nurse:

- is not afraid of complaints, recognising that they can have positive outcomes of improving future ways of working
- apologises appropriately when things go wrong, and has an adequate complaints procedure in place.

## *Stage 2: Set the standards for your outcomes*

Outcomes might include:

- the way learning is applied
- a learnt skill
- a protocol
- a strategy that is implemented
- meeting recommended standards.

- Have effective processes for preventing and managing complaints from patients in the practice.

## *Stage 3A: Identify your learning needs*

- Examine as a significant event one or more complaints, e.g. where patients have not been made aware of the complaints process.
- Compare the actual care of a patient against an acceptable standard of care for a range of clinical conditions as part of an ongoing review for a clinical area that has

been the subject of a complaint (e.g. privacy given to patients as in the case study). You could use peer review by asking respected colleagues or compare your practice against a published standard such as a guideline by a responsible body of professional opinion.

## Stage 3B: Identify your service needs

Any of the needs assessment exercises in 3A may also reveal service needs.

- Audit patient complaints in the preceding 12 months: the number, the outcomes and how the complaint system is advertised, etc.
- Audit the extent to which doctors and nurses are following practice agreed protocols. This shows how well being proactive prevents or minimises the likelihood of the source of the complaint recurring.
- Audit vulnerable areas. Look back at the analysis of complaints to identify useful areas for focusing learning, e.g. a review of the method of informing patients of the results of their cervical smears.
- Review the way that the competencies of locums are checked and that they are made aware of the practice protocols.

## Stage 4: Make and carry out a learning and action plan

- Ask your PCO to look at the practice complaints system and feed back how it can be improved (if at all).
- Arrange a tutorial with GPs, community nurses and the practice manager to discuss preventing and managing complaints.
- Undertake reflection of critical incidents including how to share the information with the practice team and respond as a team.

## Stage 5: Document your learning, competence, performance and standards of service delivery

- Collect evidence of clinical competence for all staff to guard against a complaint.
- Keep a copy of the protocol of the patient complaint process against which consecutive complaints can be audited in another 12 months' time.
- Document guidance about physical examinations including that the reason for any examination should be communicated clearly, that a chaperone should be offered for any internal or breast examination, and the comfort and privacy of the patient should always be paramount to avoid potential complaints.
- Ensure that a file containing practice protocols is available for easy reference (e.g. on the desktop of the computer).

---

**Case study 3.5 continued**

You are invited by your PCO to take part in advising practices about the handling of complaints because they were impressed by the way your complaint system was applied when you discussed this in a meeting for community nurses.

---

# References

1 Nursing and Midwifery Council (2002) *Code of Professional Conduct*. Nursing and Midwifery Council, London.

2 Chambers R and Wakley G (2000) *Making Clinical Governance Work for You*. Radcliffe Medical Press, Oxford.

3 Department of Health (2002) *Reference Guide to Consent for Examination and Treatment*. Department of Health, London. www.dh.gov.uk/assetRoot/04/01/90/61/04019061.pdf

4 The Fraser Guidelines (1985) House of Lords Judgement, London.

5 www.dh.gov.uk and enter 'research governance' into the search box for up-to-date information.

6 www.mencap.org.uk

7 Royal College of General Practitioners and Brook (2000) *Confidentiality and Young People. A toolkit for general practice, primary care groups and trusts*. Royal College of General Practitioners, London.

8 Department of Health (1997) Report of the review of patient-identifiable information. In: *The Caldicott Committee Report*. Department of Health, London. www.dh.gov.uk/assetRoot/04/06/84/04/04068404/pdf

9 Dimond B (1995) *Legal Aspects of Nursing*. Prentice Hall Nursing Series, London.

# 4

---

# Women's health and lifestyle

**Case study 4.1**

Mrs Hart comes to see you for a 'well woman' check. When you ask what prompted her to make the appointment she becomes tearful. She tells you that one of her closest friends has just had a heart attack and died. This has made her worry about the damage her own unhealthy lifestyle might be doing. You look at her – an obese woman who looks older than her 48 years, no doubt from her longstanding smoking habit. She confesses that she drinks a half or full bottle of red wine most days, rarely takes any exercise but declares that she is careful not to eat excess fat. You carry out a full health screening and give lifestyle advice, recognising that her motivation to change habits is currently high.

## What issues you should cover

### Cigarette smoking[1]

Approximately 10 million adults in the UK are cigarette smokers and a similar number are ex-smokers. The numbers of male and female smokers are about the same. More people who work in manual jobs are smokers than those employed in professional and other non-manual occupations.

About 20% of all deaths in the UK population are attributable to smoking. About half of all regular cigarette smokers will die prematurely because of their smoking habit, and a quarter of regular smokers die before the age of 70 years. It costs the NHS around £1500 million to treat patients with smoking-related diseases each year. Help Mrs Hart to understand the risks that she is running from her longstanding smoking habit – especially from lung cancer, bronchitis and emphysema and coronary heart disease – and what she has to gain from stopping smoking. About a third of deaths from cancers of all kinds can be attributed to cigarette smoking. Cigarette smoking is the most important modifiable, non-genetic, risk factor for coronary heart disease, and accounts for 11% of all heart disease deaths in women. Smoking during pregnancy is associated with an increased risk of spontaneous abortion, haemorrhage, premature birth and low birth weight as well as many problems with the infant following birth. Smoking is also associated with infertility and subfertility in women and men.

If Mrs Hart can be persuaded to stop smoking, the risks of ill-health induced by her cigarette smoking will soon fall. After one year, her risk of a heart attack will fall to about half that of a smoker; after 10 years of not smoking, her risk of lung cancer is reduced to about half that of a smoker. After 15 years of not smoking, her risk of a heart attack will be the same as if she had never smoked.

Warn Mrs Hart that when she stops smoking she may have withdrawal symptoms. These may include irritability or aggression, depression, restlessness, impaired concentration, increased appetite and craving for cigarettes. Mrs Hart may also experience light-headedness and disturbed sleep.

Psychological and behavioural techniques are key to helping patients to stop smoking. Nurses trained in supporting smoking cessation acquire skills to maintain motivation and appreciate the underlying psychology of addiction and withdrawal. The educative and supportive style of nurse consultations lends itself to interventions such as smoking cessation. Patients believe the professional information given by nurses and perceive nurses as less threatening and more approachable than doctors. Help Mrs Hart to feel that she is capable of successfully stopping smoking (self-efficacy) and how she can recognise and quash cues in her environment that will trigger cravings to smoke again. Mrs Hart's concern about her own risks from smoking following her friend's death means that health messages about stopping smoking should have a bigger impact now. Combining psychological and behavioural counselling, or group support with pharmacological interventions such as nicotine replacement or bupropion therapy, increases smoking cessation rates. Using these combination therapies, nearly one in five are still ex-smokers at six months after stopping smoking. However, longer-term follow-up studies show that many ex-smokers relapse and start smoking again. Nicotine replacement therapy is included within the *Nurse Prescribers' Formulary*.[2] Registered nurse prescribers can prescribe if they feel they have sufficient knowledge for this to fall within their 'scope of practice'.[3]

Some patients find acupuncture and hypnotherapy helpful although there is little research evidence about their effectiveness.

The six 'A's is a recommended approach for those in primary care to help patients like Mrs Hart to stop smoking.[1] That is, *ask* about smoking at every consultation, *advise* about risks and benefits of stopping smoking, *assess* patient's willingness to quit smoking, *assist* the patient in planning to stop smoking, *arrange* follow up and *audit* the practice team's success in helping patients to stop.

Many health professionals are familiar with the well known staged approach where patients are assessed for their readiness to change and smoking cessation interventions are tailored to the stage patients have reached.[4,5] Conclusions from a systematic review were that, overall, stage-based interventions are no more effective than non-stage-based interventions or no intervention, in changing smoking behaviour.[5]

Smoking is a coping mechanism for many smokers, like Mrs Hart, who may believe that cigarettes calm them down if they are worried or anxious. Many smokers will have tried unsuccessfully to give up in the past – and you will be trying to motivate Mrs Hart to quit smoking despite her feeling powerless to give up because of her past failures to do so.

# Obesity

Establish whether Mrs Hart is overweight or obese before advising her about risks to her health and treatment options. Overweight and obesity are most commonly defined by clinicians in terms of the body mass index (BMI).[6] The BMI is calculated as: weight in kg/(height in m)$^2$ and will usually be automatically calculated for you by your computer software.

Overweight is generally classed as having a BMI between 25 and 29.9 and obesity as having a BMI of 30 or over. BMI does not distinguish between mass due to body fat and muscles. Nor does it take account of the distribution of fat around the body. Some individuals who might not be defined as obese according to their BMI may still have a high degree of abdominal obesity, also termed 'central' obesity. Central obesity is measured by the waist circumference or by the waist to hip ratio. The relative distribution of fat between the waist and hip predicts subsequent coronary artery disease better than body mass index. There are increased health risks from obesity when the waist circumference exceeds 94 cm for men and 80 cm for women.[7] You will probably find that Mrs Hart has a BMI over 30 and a waist circumference of more than 80 cm if she looks obese to you.

Mrs Hart is one of many who are overweight or obese. The UK has the fastest growing rate of obesity in Europe, almost trebling in the past 20 years. Thirty-three per cent of adult women are overweight and another 20% are obese. Men have similar problems, with 45% being overweight and another 17% being obese.[8]

Ask Mrs Hart if she indulges in 'binge eating' – a pattern that may be present in 20–30% of people who are obese. Binge eating is eating an amount of food that is larger than most people would eat in a similar time under similar circumstances. Ask about her typical food intake – does she accept she is eating too much, or is physically inactive? It is common for obese and overweight people to underestimate their food intake by about a third – perhaps because of genuine forgetfulness or self-deception or a lack of understanding of food composition, particularly hidden fat. In particular, people under-report their eating of snacks when they are totting up what they have eaten in a day.

Warn Mrs Hart about the risks to her health from her obesity. Obesity leads to premature mortality – there are lots of facts given in Tables 4.1 and 4.2 that you can relay to Mrs Hart. For instance, the risk of a fatal or non-fatal myocardial infarction among women with a BMI greater than 29 is three times that of lean women after adjustment for age and smoking.[9] Table 4.1 lists the proportion of various health problems that can be attributed to overweight or obesity. Mrs Hart might be impressed by the figures for the relative risks she is running of diabetes, hypertension, myocardial infarction and other clinical conditions compared with a woman who is not obese – try quoting some of the statistics listed in Table 4.2 to her.

Tell Mrs Hart about the likely benefits to her health from losing weight. Specific examples can be impressive. For instance, in one study of 1200 people whose BMIs were between 25 and 37 and none of whom were being treated for hypertension, those who had lost at least 4.5 kg of weight by six months had an initial average fall in systolic and diastolic blood pressures of 8 or 9 mmHg that was maintained at follow up 36 months later. The lower levels of blood pressure at six months were not

**Table 4.1:**   Proportion of various conditions attributable to excess weight (BMI $> 27$ kg/m$^2$)[9]

| Disease | Number out of 100 people |
|---|---|
| Hypertension | 24.1 |
| Myocardial infarction | 13.9 |
| Angina pectoris | 20.5 |
| Stroke | 25.8 |
| Venous thrombosis | 7.7 |
| Type 2 diabetes | 24.1 |
| Hyperlipidaemia | 7.7 |
| Gout | 20.0 |
| Osteoarthritis | 11.8 |
| Gall bladder disease | 14.3 |
| Colorectal cancer | 4.7 |
| Breast cancer | 3.2 |
| Genitourinary cancer | 9.1 |

**Table 4.2:**   Relative risks of different health problems in obese versus non-obese people[8]

| Condition | Relative risk | |
|---|---|---|
| | Women | Men |
| Type 2 diabetes | 12.7 | 5.2 |
| Hypertension | 4.2 | 2.6 |
| Heart attack | 3.2 | 1.5 |
| Colon cancer | 2.7 | 3.0 |
| Angina | 1.8 | 1.8 |
| Gall bladder disease | 1.8 | 1.8 |
| Ovarian cancer | 1.7 | |
| Osteoarthritis | 1.4 | 1.9 |
| Stroke | 1.3 | 1.3 |

*Obesity = BMI $> 30$ kg/m$^2$*
*The risk for a non-obese person is taken as 1 and the relative risk of an obese person developing the conditions is given in comparison for men and women.*

maintained at follow up in those who failed to sustain the 4.5 kg or more weight loss at six months.[10] There is now consistent evidence that weight loss not only reduces blood pressure in people who are overweight and hypertensive, but also in those who are overweight with high-normal blood pressure.

A 10% loss of body weight over the course of one year is a realistic target for most people. Box 4.1 describes the range of benefits to Mrs Hart's health she could expect if she lost 10% of her body weight in the next 12 months.

Mrs Hart may ask for advice about diet. There has been a great deal of recent interest in the efficacy of low carbohydrate diets. A systematic review concluded that there was insufficient evidence to make recommendations for or against the use of low carbohydrate diets. Weight loss among obese people was associated with longer diet duration and decreased calorie intake rather than the carbohydrate content of their diet. Low carbohydrate diets appeared to have no significant adverse effects on serum lipids, fasting glucose or insulin levels or blood pressure in one study.[11] Another reviewer concluded that the choice of diet

> may come down to suitably matching a dietary regimen to an individual's taste. For some of us a high protein diet with bacon and eggs, steak, fish and cheese would be heaven. For others, purgatory. Perhaps now people who want or need to lose weight have more of a choice about what might best suit them.[12]

---

**Box 4.1:**  Benefits of 10% loss of body weight in an obese person[13]

**Mortality**
- More than 20% decrease in premature mortality
- More than 30% decrease in diabetes related deaths

**Blood pressure**
- 10 mmHg decrease in systolic BP
- 20 mmHg decrease in diastolic BP

**Diabetes**
- 50% decrease in fasting glucose

**Lipids**
- 30% decrease in triglycerides
- 10% decrease in total cholesterol
- 15% decrease in low density lipoprotein (LDL) cholesterol
- 8% increase in high density lipoprotein (HDL) cholesterol

---

Many nurses working in primary care run successful weight control groups. These can be time-effective as a nurse can give more patients attention and education within an hour-long group than he or she could support if seeing them individually. A group atmosphere can also provide peer support and help to alleviate the feelings of isolation and low self-esteem that frequently accompany obesity.

Mrs Hart may feel that she cannot lose weight without additional help and ask about drug therapy. Consider drug treatment as a second choice option, with the initial interventions being targeted on behaviour change. If patients opt for drug treatment (from a fully informed perspective), combine this with diet and behaviour management in a partnership approach.

Patients should show that they are motivated by losing at least 2.5 kg over a four-week period before being prescribed drug treatment.

Drug therapy available to obese patients includes:

* orlistat (Xenical) which decreases fat absorption by inhibiting the enzyme lipase
* sibutramine (Reductil), a serotonin and noradrenaline re-uptake inhibitor.

You will need to be able to explain to Mrs Hart the advantages and disadvantages of drug therapy and the commitment she will be making to maintaining weight loss through dietary control and increased physical activity. Nurses who are registered as supplementary prescribers with the NMC can prescribe drugs for obesity if the independent medical practitioner agrees, using a clinical management plan.[14] Use medication as an adjunct to dietary, lifestyle and behavioural therapies in patients with sufficient motivation to adhere to an appropriate dietary regime.

Criteria for prescribing orlistat in line with NICE guidelines are given in Box 4.2. Orlistat is used in conjunction with a mildly hypocaloric diet containing around a third of calories from fat. Orlistat has an optimum effect at a dose of 120 mg three times a day. It is taken before, during or up to an hour after each main meal and the dose is omitted if a meal is missed or contains no fat.[15] Adverse effects such as oily spotting from the rectum, flatulence and faecal urgency occur in up to 27% of people taking orlistat.[16]

---

**Box 4.2:**   Criteria for prescribing orlistat[17]

* The licensing criteria and the NICE recommendations require potential patients to lose 2.5 kg in the month preceding the first prescription for orlistat, by dietary control and increased physical activity. This indicates whether a person is able to maintain a suitably low fat intake and reasonable amount of physical activity.
* Patients should have documented evidence of a BMI of 30 and above or a BMI of 28 and above with significant co-morbidity such as type 2 diabetes, hypertension or dyslipidaemia.
* Patients taking orlistat should be offered specific concomitant advice, support and counselling on diet, physical activity and behavioural strategies.
* People taking orlistat should be monitored and weighed on a monthly basis and thereafter as part of a supervised weight management plan.
* People continuing to be prescribed orlistat should have 5% weight loss at three months from the start of drug treatment and at least 10% cumulative weight loss at six months from the start of treatment.
* Treatment should not be continued beyond 12 months, and never beyond 24 months.
* The medication can only be prescribed for adults aged 18 to 75 years old.

---

NICE guidance is similar in recommending that sibutramine should only be prescribed for people who have seriously attempted to lose weight by diet, exercise and other behavioural modifications, and those prescribed the drug should be offered specific support, advice and counselling on these factors.[17,18] Sibutramine should only be used for people in the same category of risk from their overweight or obesity as for orlistat (*see* Box 4.2). Sibutramine creates a feeling of satiety by acting as a sero-tonin and noradrenaline re-uptake inhibitor in the brain, enabling patients to feel satisfied after eating smaller quantities of food. It may also increase thermogenesis by stimulant action on the peripheral noradrenergic system. Monitoring of treatment is essential (*see* Box 4.3). Weight loss is maximal over the first six months and continues at a slower rate thereafter.[19] Sibutramine can reduce total cholesterol and triglycerides, with an increase in HDL cholesterol, and improved glycaemic control in type 2 diabetes.[20] Serious adverse effects include a rise in blood pressure, and pulmonary hypertension. Less serious side-effects include headache, dry mouth, anorexia, constipation, insomnia, rhinitis, and pharyngitis in up to 30% of people taking sibutramine.[16]

---

**Box 4.3:** Monitoring treatment for sibutramine

- Monitor pulse and blood pressure every two weeks for three months then monthly until six months. Keep monitoring regularly thereafter.
- Monitor for signs of pulmonary hypertension.
- Encourage healthy sensible eating patterns and increased regular exercise.
- Weigh at each review attendance.
- Start on 10 mg once daily.
- If weight loss is less than 2 kg after four weeks, increase to 15 mg per day.
- Then, if weight loss is less than 2 kg over a four-week period on the higher dose, discontinue.
- The maximum period of treatment is one year.

---

Screening Mrs Hart for depression and anxiety may be worthwhile, as psychological factors have been shown to be major predictors of weight gain in middle aged women.[21]

## Reducing dietary fat

Mrs Hart already claimed that she minimises fat in her diet. Less total fat or less of any individual fatty acid fraction in the diet is beneficial. A reduction of over 20% in total serum cholesterol concentration can result in a corresponding 25% fall in mortality from coronary heart disease.[8]

A recent systematic review of trials of diets that modified or reduced fat intake for at least six months has concluded that there is a:

small but potentially important reduction in cardiovascular risk with reduction or modification of dietary fat intake, seen particularly in trials of longer duration.[22]

There were reductions in cardiovascular events of up to 24% in trials lasting for at least two years, but it was not clear whether it was the duration of the intervention, or the length of follow up that was critical in determining whether the intervention was effective. However, there was little effect on total mortality.[22]

## Physical activity

Mrs Hart may not be sure what type of physical activity she could try if she has led a sedentary life recently. Tell her that good advice is to:

> try to build up gradually to take half an hour of moderate intensity physical activity on five or more days of the week. Activities like brisk walking, cycling, swimming, dancing and gardening are good options.[23]

Warn Mrs Hart that physical inactivity doubles the risk of coronary heart disease, is a major risk factor for stroke and contributes to the increased frequency of overweight and obesity. There is a graded inverse relationship between physical activity and the risk of coronary events occurring.

In the general UK population, only a third of men (33%) and a fifth of women (21%) meet the current guidelines for physical activity – of moderate or vigorous activity for at least 30 minutes at a time, on five or more days a week.

Nurses working in primary care are ideally placed to set up exercise groups within the community. These could be established after seeking advice from physiotherapist colleagues, and may comprise simple exercise such as fast walking. Middle aged or elderly patients may be more likely to attend this sort of low key approach rather than attending a gym or a fitness centre where they anticipate that they will feel out of place.

## Alcohol

Alcohol has nearly as much energy as fat at 7 kcal/g. It can compromise a weight-reducing diet, providing hidden calories. It is thought to alter the pattern of fat distribution encouraging a 'beer belly'. Excessive amounts of alcohol act as a central depressant and sap initiative and will power, reducing enthusiasm for physical exercise. Mrs Hart has already admitted to drinking excessive alcohol – a half to a full bottle of wine per day, which probably add up to an average four or five units of alcohol per day and more than 30 units of alcohol per week. The government recommends that women should drink no more than two to three units of alcohol per day and men three to four units of alcohol per day, as women are more sensitive to the adverse effects of alcohol than men.[24]

It is widely believed that drinking red wine is good for the heart, but this benefit has only been shown to apply to those groups at risk of coronary heart disease – men over 40 years and post-menopausal women – and is at its greatest benefit between one and two units of alcohol per day (all forms of alcohol and not just red wine).[24]

Around one-fifth of adults attending primary care are heavy drinkers – their drinking is generally missed by their GPs even though studies have shown that problem drinkers consult their GPs twice as often as other patients.[25] People do not usually seek help for their alcohol problems directly but present with other complaints such as dyspepsia, sleeplessness, heart arrhythmias or psychosocial problems. Early detection of and counselling in alcohol misuse, by primary care doctors as a brief alcohol intervention, is known to be effective but many health professionals seem to consider that the drinking of alcohol is part of a patient's private life that should not be invaded if it is not presented as a problem.[26,27]

The simplest way to detect heavy drinking is to ask the person about their alcohol consumption – how much and how often. You could use the CAGE questionnaire where two or more positive answers suggests that the patient has a problem with alcohol:

- have you ever felt you ought to **C**ut down on your drinking?
- have people **A**nnoyed you by criticising your drinking?
- have you ever felt bad or **G**uilty about your drinking?
- have you ever had a drink first thing in the morning (**E**ye-opener) to steady your nerves or get rid of a hangover?

A good approach to take with Mrs Hart will be to spend five minutes with her now or at another appointment discussing the costs, risks and benefits from her perspective. Emphasise that she needs to reduce or stop her alcohol intake. Discuss with her what further support the practice or other agencies can offer.[28] Although there is no reliable laboratory marker for the effects of excessive alcohol consumption, you could arrange blood tests to see if the mean corpuscular volume is raised or liver function tests abnormal – an isolated or disproportionately high gamma glutamyl transpeptidase (GGT) may be due to liver enzyme induction caused by alcohol, but could also be caused by other drugs such as phenytoin.

## Sexual health and cervical screening

A well woman check should incorporate a review of Mrs Hart's sexual health. A sexual health history fits in well with enquiries made about general health and lifestyle. You would not, of course, fall into the trap of making assumptions from Mrs Hart's appearance that she is, or has not been, exposed to sexual health risks! You will need to enquire about whether Mrs Hart has a current partner, if she is sexually active with this partner, and how long she has been with this partner. This can lead into a past history of changes of partnerships to give an estimation of her risk of acquiring sexually transmitted infections. Remember not to make assumptions that a patient is with a partner currently, or that any partnership is heterosexual.

Approximately 3000 new cases of cervical cancer are diagnosed each year in England and Wales, leading to about 1200 deaths.[29] About half of the women who present with late stage cervical cancer have never had a cervical smear. The presence of human papilloma virus (HPV) types 16 and 18 (and less commonly some of the other types of HPV) has been shown to be associated with the development of cervical cancer. The risk of acquiring HPV increases with having larger numbers of sexual partners, or a partner who has had many previous sexual partners.

The current cervical screening test is based on taking a sample of cells from the cervix with a wooden or plastic shaped spatula. The material collected is spread on a glass slide and sprayed with fixative. Specially trained cytologists examine the slide for abnormal cells. Relatively high numbers of slides are inadequate for examination because the cells are obscured by debris or blood, or are too thick or thin. Fatigue by cytologists is a significant cause of failure to avoid false negative or false positive results. The newer liquid-based cytology has a much lower rate of inadequate slides and clearer, more easily read slides with the potential for automated slide examination. The sample is collected from the cervix in the same way, but using a special plastic broom-like device which is swept over the transitional zone five times to collect cellular material. The broom is rinsed in a vial of preservative. The vial is mixed in the laboratory and treated to remove unwanted material by an automated process. The remaining suspension of cells can be stained and the prepared slide looks much clearer for examination. The automation of the slide examination is also under trial. The proportion of inadequate smears (and subsequent repeat tests required) is greatly reduced.[30]

You might need to explain to Mrs Hart that cervical screening at between three and five year intervals provides the best chance of picking up abnormal cells. Decreasing the interval to less than three years increases the pick-up rate only slightly in those with a previous negative test. Most authorities suggest that screening should be every three years initially until two or three negative results have been obtained, then five yearly. Recommendations that are in the process of being implemented are to start screening at three yearly intervals from the age of 25 years of age, and to switch to five yearly intervals after the age of 49 years of age, discontinuing screening at 64 years of age in people who have had negative tests.[31]

---

**Case study 4.1 continued**

Mrs Hart is not sure that she can give up smoking while she still feels so distressed over her friend's heart attack, but decides to go to the local leisure centre to enrol on an exercise programme. When she attends for her routine cervical smear, she tells you that the regular exercise helps to relax her so that she drinks less and she has started to reduce her smoking as well.

---

# Collecting data to demonstrate your learning, competence, performance and standards of service delivery

## Example cycle of evidence 4.1

- Focus: clinical care
- Other relevant focus: smoking cessation

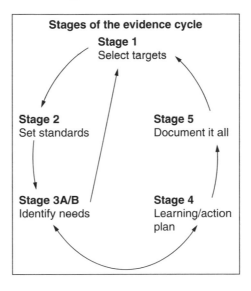

**Stages of the evidence cycle**

**Stage 1**
Select targets

**Stage 2**
Set standards

**Stage 5**
Document it all

**Stage 3A/B**
Identify needs

**Stage 4**
Learning/action plan

---

**Case study 4.2**

Miss Flower has just had her first baby. At five pounds the baby was small for a full-term baby. Miss Flower is a smoker and she tells you that apart from the midwife mentioning that she should stop smoking when she first booked in for her pregnancy, no one else has ever advised her to stop smoking in the past when she has come for contraceptive or other healthcare.

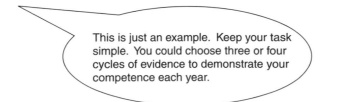

This is just an example. Keep your task simple. You could choose three or four cycles of evidence to demonstrate your competence each year.

*Stage 1: Select your aspirations for good practice*

The excellent nurse has:

- a structured approach for managing long-term health problems and preventive care.

*Stage 2: Set the standards for your outcomes*

Outcomes might include:

- the way learning is applied
- a learnt skill
- a protocol
- a strategy that is implemented
- meeting recommended standards.

- Every patient attending for antenatal care in the first trimester or for contraceptive care is asked if they smoke and has their smoking history recorded.
- All pregnant women who smoke are offered advice about the risks of smoking and the benefits of quitting, and further support and help.

*Stage 3A: Identify your learning needs*

- Self-assess your knowledge of the magnitude and nature of health risks associated with women who are smokers and especially those who are pregnant.
- Carry out a patient survey: ask 10 consecutive patients who smoke (some should be pregnant) if they have received advice about smoking within the previous two years, and if so, how appropriate the advice was perceived to be, when it had been given and by whom.

*Stage 3B: Identify your service needs*

Any of the needs assessment exercises in 3A may also reveal service needs.

- Audit the smoking status of patients attending antenatal care in the last trimester for: existence of record of smoking status, extent of advice and support or help offered, and the change of smoking behaviour at the postnatal appointment.
- Carry out a significant event audit of cases of babies born to mothers who smoke who have health problems that might be associated with mother's smoking status, e.g. low birth weight, ear and chest infections in the first 12 months.

## Stage 4: Make and carry out a learning and action plan

- Read up about risks of smoking and provision of best practice in motivating people to stop smoking.
- Talk to smokers at an informal group, e.g. in the waiting room during antenatal clinic, and actively listen to their feedback about improving services and the quality and extent of the advice they have received about stopping smoking.
- Audiotape (with the patient's informed consent) a consultation (or two) where you give advice to a patient who is a smoker, offer them further help and try to motivate them to stop. Ask a health promotion expert to comment on your approach and give targeted feedback to you about your knowledge, skills and attitudes.

## Stage 5: Document your learning, competence, performance and standards of service delivery

- Keep the surveys of smokers – two separate cohorts of patients at different time periods before and after putting your learning and action plan into practice, or one cohort of the same patients surveyed twice over time.
- Keep a copy of the practice protocol relating to smoking cessation.
- Carry out a re-audit of the recording in antenatal patients' notes of smoking status, extent of advice and support or help offered, and the change of smoking behaviour at follow up.

---

**Case study 4.2 continued**

Miss Flower's baby thrives as she makes up her mind not to inflict passive smoking on her baby or her partner at home. She quits after only using nicotine replacement therapy for a month and had not resumed smoking 12 months later.

---

# Example cycle of evidence 4.2

- Focus: probity
- Other relevant focus: smoking cessation

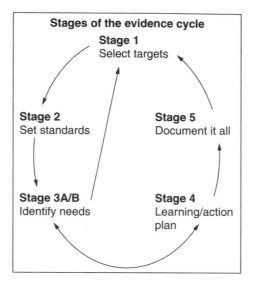

Stages of the evidence cycle

**Stage 1**
Select targets

**Stage 2**
Set standards

**Stage 5**
Document it all

**Stage 3A/B**
Identify needs

**Stage 4**
Learning/action plan

---

**Case study 4.3**

In an external inspection by the Healthcare Commission, the reviewers note that patient-identifiable information about smoking cessation is being passed to the PCT to trigger payments to practices without proper accountability. You are asked to clarify the role of community nurses, GPs, administrative staff and healthcare assistants in regard to smoking cessation, and ascertain who takes responsibility for passing on information to the PCT and that there is a clear audit trail to follow.

This is just an example. Keep your task simple. You could choose three or four cycles of evidence to demonstrate your competence each year.

## Stage 1: Select your aspirations for good practice

The excellent nurse:

- ensures that health promotion activities such as smoking cessation have a defined audit pathway of which all professionals are aware
- has effective systems in the practice so that all team members understand their personal and collective responsibilities for the care and safety of patients.

## Stage 2: Set the standards for your outcomes

> Outcomes might include:
>
> - the way learning is applied
> - a learnt skill
> - a protocol
> - a strategy that is implemented
> - meeting recommended standards.

- Compose and agree standards and processes for the way in which health professionals take responsibility for offering, providing and claiming for undertaking smoking cessation services.

## Stage 3A: Identify your learning needs

- Reflect on how lines of responsibility work in the practice team, including how sure you are about who should do what and who takes responsibility for opportunistic and systematic advice to patients who smoke.

## Stage 3B: Identify your service needs

> Any of the needs assessment exercises in 3A may also reveal service needs.

- Review the practice protocols for line management and accountability with the practice team in respect of all aspects of smoking cessation services. You should look for gaps and inconsistencies and include staff knowledge and skills, resources and promotional literature, finance claims and complaints.
- Draw up a table that identifies the level of expertise in smoking cessation that exists for each community nurse, GP and allied health professional attached to the practice. Circulate this within the team so that team members can identify their own level, and when completed distribute it to all team members so that there is awareness of each other's skills.
- The development needs of staff should become apparent and this may also enable you to see if in-house training can be provided from the 'experts' within your team.

*Stage 4: Make and carry out a learning and action plan*

- Attend relevant clinical management workshops. Lobby the PCT to provide these if they are not currently available.
- Update the practice protocol for smoking cessation to address gaps and inconsistencies identified in section 3B. Discuss at team meetings.
- Read the job evaluation handbook to understand what levels of knowledge and skills and other qualities team members should have.[32]

*Stage 5: Document your learning, competence, performance and standards of service delivery*

- Record the revised practice protocols clarifying lines of responsibility.
- Keep a copy of the table depicting levels of expertise across the entire practice team enabling appropriate use of each other's skills.
- Record the smoking cessation services undertaken by all health professionals attached to a practice – with no patient-identifiable information.

---

**Case study 4.3 continued**

You have audited how all the clinical and non-clinical members of the practice team manage smoking cessation using a revised protocol with which the whole team is familiar. You now consider how this global team approach to preventive services could be generalised to other areas of practice.

---

# Example cycle of evidence 4.3

- Focus: maintaining good medical practice
- Other relevant focus: management of obesity

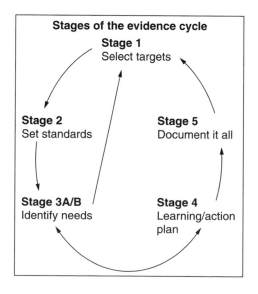

**Stages of the evidence cycle**

**Stage 1**
Select targets

**Stage 2**
Set standards

**Stage 5**
Document it all

**Stage 3A/B**
Identify needs

**Stage 4**
Learning/action plan

**Case study 4.4**

When Mrs Chubb got promotion she found that she was nervous about giving talks to groups of people and realised that her self-confidence was undermined by her obesity. After trying to lose weight herself with some success, she has come to you for help. She tells you that she has a friend who is receiving slimming tablets on prescription and wonders whether you feel the doctor would prescribe these for her.

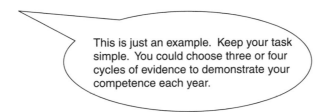

This is just an example. Keep your task simple. You could choose three or four cycles of evidence to demonstrate your competence each year.

## *Stage 1: Select your aspirations for good practice*

The excellent nurse:

- is up to date with developments in clinical practice and regularly reviews her knowledge and performance
- communicates well with medical colleagues in order to provide consistency of approach.

## *Stage 2: Set the standards for your outcomes*

Outcomes might include:

- the way learning is applied
- a learnt skill
- a protocol
- a strategy that is implemented
- meeting recommended standards.

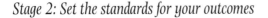

- An audit of the prescribing of anti-obesity medications within the practice demonstrates that clinical performance is in line with NICE guidance.
- Data from audits show that patients attending the weight control clinic do at least as well as in other general practices.

## Stage 3A: Identify your learning needs

- Record entries in your reflective diary when overweight or obese patients request anti-obesity drugs. Consider how sure you are about the NICE guidelines about which patients may receive orlistat or sibutramine.
- Survey 10 consecutive patients whom you have advised about their weight. Ask them if they consider that you are good at explaining options and best practice to them as patients.
- Record any unsolicited or requested comments from the rest of the practice team about your management of patients with obesity.

## Stage 3B: Identify your service needs

Any of the needs assessment exercises in 3A may also reveal service needs.

- Compare the audit of your weight control clinic with clinics run in neighbouring practices and talk to colleagues about the way in which they run their clinics in comparison to yours.
- Record how the practice team deals with protests or other negative comments from patients denied anti-obesity drugs. This should be because they are outside NICE guidelines e.g. their BMI is too low, they have lost too little weight to justify starting an anti-obesity drug or the time limit for prescribing has expired.
- Organise a patient survey to determine the quality of information on weight management given by all members of the practice team.

## Stage 4: Make and carry out a learning and action plan

- Arrange to meet with a local dietician to gain information on running a weight control clinic and discuss topics and resources that would be useful.
- Download and read NICE guidance relating to prescribing of anti-obesity drugs.
- Talk to obese patients and listen to their perspectives about adverse effects/benefits of anti-obesity drugs.
- Compose a practice protocol with contributions from the whole primary care team as part of an in-house educational meeting.
- Audit the change in weight of overweight/obese patients over a 12-month period, whether or not they have received anti-obesity drugs. Flag their notes on computer screens so that successive GPs and practice nurses monitor their weight. Compare your audits with the results from other general practices.

## Stage 5: Document your learning, competence, performance and standards of service delivery

- Keep written reflections on your gain in knowledge and skills.

- Conduct a re-audit of treatment of obese patients against NICE guidance and the practice protocol, and enclose your revised protocol.
- Record the findings of the patient survey, including of obese patients, about the quality of information given about weight management.
- Record the comparison of your audits of your clinics with the results from other general practices.

---

**Case study 4.4 continued**

The GP agreed that Mrs Chubb should receive orlistat because the course of medication was justified according to NICE criteria. She has managed to lose two stone in weight over the following 12 months while she also attended your weight control clinic. However, she stopped attending the clinic and started to regain the weight in the first six months when she was not taking orlistat.

---

# Example cycle of evidence 4.4

- Focus: maintaining good medical practice
- Other relevant focus: managing patients who drink excessive alcohol

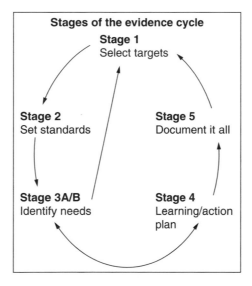

Stages of the evidence cycle

Stage 1
Select targets

Stage 2
Set standards

Stage 5
Document it all

Stage 3A/B
Identify needs

Stage 4
Learning/action plan

**Case study 4.5**

Mrs Mellow has been going to see her GP in the practice frequently over the past year with minor complaints such as dyspepsia, irritability and difficulties getting to sleep. The GP refers her to you to undertake a 'general health screening' in an attempt to get to the root of this problem. Mrs Mellow arrives late for her appointment. Whilst checking her blood pressure you notice that her breath smells of alcohol, and you wonder if this is the cause behind her frequent consultations. You are unsure how to challenge her about this assumption and feel that you need to find out how to do this.

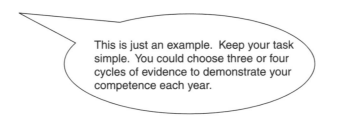

This is just an example. Keep your task simple. You could choose three or four cycles of evidence to demonstrate your competence each year.

*Stage 1: Select your aspirations for good practice*

The excellent nurse:

• makes sound management decisions, which are based on good practice and evidence.

*Stage 2: Set the standards for your outcomes*

Outcomes might include:

• the way learning is applied
• a learnt skill
• a protocol
• a strategy that is implemented
• meeting recommended standards.

• You and all other members of the primary care team are skilled in the recognition and management of people who drink excessive alcohol.

*Stage 3A: Identify your learning needs*

• Write down the four questions from the CAGE questionnaire and check to see if you have remembered them correctly so that you can pose them to patients (*see* page 63).

- Ask patients to complete an exit questionnaire about their lifestyle habits as they leave after a consultation with anyone in the team. They can complete it in the surgery and leave it in a secure collection box at reception. Compare this with the records about smoking, alcohol and exercise habits in their medical notes.

## Stage 3B: Identify your service needs

> Any of the needs assessment exercises in 3A may also reveal service needs.

- Organise a SCOT analysis of recognition and management of patients who have excessive alcohol intake. You might discuss this in a team meeting.
- Visit a neighbouring practice known for the well co-ordinated way they manage lifestyle screening and preventive care of those with problems from heavy drinking.
- Review the patient literature relating to limits on alcohol consumption to see if it is in date and appropriate for your patient population. Consider putting together differing information packs which are applicable to a variety of age groups.
- Contact the local community substance abuse nurse and ask if they can come to a staff meeting to talk about how the team could be more active in their attempts to identify heavy drinkers.
- Undertake a training needs analysis for you and the practice team. Ascertain any gaps between expected and actual levels of knowledge and skills in relation to recognising and managing patients who are heavy drinkers of alcohol. The local community substance abuse nurse may be able to help you with this.

## Stage 4: Make and carry out a learning and action plan

- Organise a 'how to do it' workshop on the national recommendations for alcohol intake and the carrying out of brief interventions in primary care. Ask a health promotion expert to run it as an in-house event for all the practice team.
- Write a short newsletter for patients describing lifestyle interventions (including alcohol) available at the practice and through other agencies.
- Plan to address challenges and opportunities that have emerged from the SCOT analysis. Make changes such as in the way care is delivered or how information about alcohol is recorded or how the team communicates.

## Stage 5: Document your learning, competence, performance and standards of service delivery

- Keep a copy of the training needs analysis of you and the practice team in relation to section 3B above.
- Keep a copy of your PDP recording the gaps in your knowledge and skills and completion of your learning plan.

- Keep records of the SCOT analysis and the plan to address challenges and opportunities in relation to recognition and management of patients (and staff) with alcohol problems.

---

**Case study 4.5 continued**

Mrs Mellow's son is home from university and comes to see you complaining of dyspepsia, irritability and difficulties with sleep. You ask him about his lifestyle and smoking and drinking habits. You pose the four questions in the CAGE questionnaire. He is surprised that you think his regular intake of three or four pints of beer a day might be the cause of his complaints as he feels he drinks a lot less than his mates. He agrees to reduce his drinking for a trial period and to come and see you again in a few weeks' time.

---

## Example cycle of evidence 4.5

- Focus: relationships with patients
- Other relevant focus: health promotion by yourself and the practice team

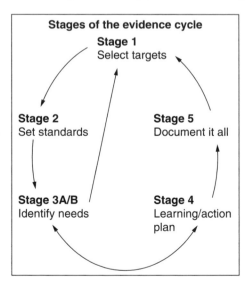

**Stages of the evidence cycle**

**Stage 1**
Select targets

**Stage 2**
Set standards

**Stage 3A/B**
Identify needs

**Stage 4**
Learning/action plan

**Stage 5**
Document it all

---

**Case study 4.6**

As Mrs Test neared her 50th birthday she wanted a full 'MOT' to check that she had no health problems. She contacted the surgery to see if she could book in for a well woman check. She explained that she just wanted a mammogram and blood tests. She added that she could do without the lecture she knew she would get about smoking and lack of exercise.

---

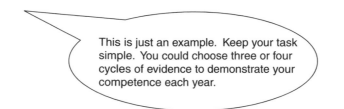

This is just an example. Keep your task simple. You could choose three or four cycles of evidence to demonstrate your competence each year.

## Stage 1: Select your aspirations for good practice

The excellent nurse:

- gives patients the information they need about their problem in a way they can understand
- respects the right of patients to refuse treatments or tests.

## Stage 2: Set the standards for your outcomes

Outcomes might include:

- the way learning is applied
- a learnt skill
- a protocol
- a strategy that is implemented
- meeting recommended standards.

- The practice has an up-to-date protocol for a well woman clinic individualised for age groups of women.
- The practice has a bank of health promotion literature and other resources linked to the processes undertaken in the well woman clinic.

## Stage 3A: Identify your learning needs

- Issue anonymised comment slips to the next 10 consecutive female patients who attend the well woman clinic or book in for a health promotion check with you.
- You and the reception staff keep notes of direct feedback from individual patients about any aspect of health promotion or lifestyle advice and look for trends or patterns.
- Consider if you are competent to give patients up-to-date information and balanced advice about the risks and benefits of screening, for example, breast screening for women in their forties, bone density scanning for those with a family history of osteoporosis, or cervical cytology for those in their late fifties who have always had normal cervical smears.

## Stage 3B: Identify your service needs

> Any of the needs assessment exercises in 3A may also reveal service needs.

- Compare the views of different types of patients, if it is clear from the comment slips (as above in section 3A) that they are different, e.g. women living in inner cities or in rural communities, or women in employment or not employed, or by socio-economic characteristics as appropriate.
- Undertake a significant event audit with key members of the practice team of e.g. a woman who presents with a stroke in her late fifties and who has never had her blood pressure recorded in her notes.
- Audiotape (with patients' informed consent) yourself giving health promotion advice. Swap tapes with colleagues and peer review for style of communication and content.

## Stage 4: Make and carry out a learning and action plan

- Attend an update lecture on screening and ask the experts questions about risks and benefits of screening as posed in section 3A above. Write down the answers to reflect on later.
- Study the feedback from patients and reflect on how to make changes to meet the needs of patients more effectively. Revise the protocol for the well woman clinic accordingly in discussion with the practice team.
- Read the manufacturers' literature that patients receive with nicotine replacement and anti-obesity therapy and other health promotion literature you have been distributing to patients, so that you know what information patients may be reading.
- Revise the 'well woman check' protocol with other team members and plan an audit to monitor its use.
- After obtaining the feedback from patients, write a service improvement plan.

## Stage 5: Document your learning, competence, performance and standards of service delivery

- Write a list of the frequently asked questions from patients and the answers and distribute it to the whole healthcare team in an attempt to improve the consistency of advice when giving health promotion.
- Include in your portfolio a copy of the service improvement plan.
- Keep a list of the packs of information that are suited to differing ages and needs.
- Include a copy of the 'well woman check' protocol.
- Keep the peer review on the audiotaped consultations. Plan to arrange for another peer review exchange in about two years to check on your competence.

---

**Case study 4.6 continued**

Mrs Test attends for a 'well person' check. You ask how she feels about being a smoker and not taking any exercise. Mrs Test states that she is happy with her lifestyle as she doesn't believe in exercise and has no intention to stop smoking even though she knows it's bad for her. However, when you discuss Mrs Test's weight she immediately tells you that she is not happy with her size and is anxious to lose weight. You therefore proceed to give plentiful advice on dietary changes and how exercise would help with weight loss, recognising that this is where her motivation is currently high. You act in partnership with her to make this a priority area for changes in health behaviour.

---

# References

1   Munafo M, Drury M, Wakley G, Chambers R and Murphy M (2003) *Smoking Cessation Matters in Primary Care*. Radcliffe Medical Press, Oxford.

2   Joint Formulary Committee (2003) *Nurse Prescribers' Formulary 2003–2004*. British Medical Association and Royal Pharmaceutical Society of Great Britain, London.

3   Nursing and Midwifery Council (2002) *Code of Professional Conduct*. Nursing and Midwifery Council, London.

4   Prochaska JO, DiClemente CC and Norcross JC (1992) In search of how people change. Applications to addictive behaviours. *The American Psychologist*. **47**: 1102–14.

5   Riemsma RP, Pattenden J, Bridle C *et al.* (2003) Systematic review of the effectiveness of stage based interventions to promote smoking cessation. *British Medical Journal*. **326**: 1175–7.

6   Chambers R and Wakley G (2002) *Obesity and Overweight Matters in Primary Care*. Radcliffe Medical Press, Oxford.

7   World Health Organization (1997) *Obesity: preventing and managing the global epidemic*. World Health Organization, Geneva.

8   National Audit Office (2001) *Tackling Obesity in England*. National Audit Office, London.

9   Garrow J (2000) Health risks of obesity. In: *Report of the British Nutrition Foundation Task Force. Obesity*. British Nutrition Foundation, Blackwell Science, Oxford.

10  Stevens V, Obarzanek E, Cook N *et al.* (2001) Long-term weight loss and changes in blood pressure: results of the trials of hypertension prevention, Phase II. *Annals of Internal Medicine*. **134**: 1–11.

11  Bravata DM, Sanders L, Huang J *et al.* (2003) Efficacy and safety of low-carbohydrate diets. *Journal of the American Medical Association*. **289(14)**: 1837–49.

12  Moore A and McQuay H (eds) (2003) Low carbohydrate diets – two RCTs and a systematic review. *Bandolier 113*. **10(2)**: 4–5.

13  Maryon Davis A, Giles A and Rona R (2000) *Tackling Obesity: a toolbox for local partnership action*. Faculty of Public Health, Royal College of Physicians of the UK, London.

14  Department of Health (2003) *Implementation Guide to Extended and Supplementary Nurse Prescribing*. Department of Health, London.

15  Joint Formulary Committee (2004) *British National Formulary*. British Medical Association and Royal Pharmaceutical Society of Great Britain, London.

16  Godlee F (ed.) (2004) *Clinical Evidence Concise*. Issue 11. BMJ Publishing Group, London.

17  National Institute for Clinical Excellence (2001) *Guidance on the Use of Orlistat for the Treatment of Obesity in Adults*. National Institute for Clinical Excellence, London.

18  National Institute for Clinical Excellence (2001) *Guidance on the Use of Sibutramine for the Treatment of Obesity in Adults*. National Institute for Clinical Excellence, London.

19  Apfelbaum M, Vague P, Ziegler O *et al.* (1999) Long-term maintenance of weight loss after a very low calorie diet: a randomised trial of the efficacy and tolerability of sibutramine. *Americal Journal of Medicine.* **106**: 179–84.

20  Sjostrum L, Rissanen A, Andersen T *et al.* for the European Multicentre Orlistat Study Group (2000) Randomized double blind placebo controlled multicenter study of sibutramine in obese hypertensive patients. *Cardiology.* **94**: 152–8.

21  Sammel MD, Grisso JA, Freeman EW *et al.* (2003) Weight gain among women in the late reproductive years. *Family Practice.* **20**: 401–9.

22  Hooper L, Summerbell C, Higgins J *et al.* (2001) Dietary fat intake and prevention of cardiovascular disease: systematic review. *British Medical Journal.* **322**: 757–63.

23  Health Education Authority (1998) *Managing Weight. A workbook for health and other professionals*. Health Education Authority, London.

24  Waller S and Naidoo B (2002) Prevention and Reduction of Alcohol Misuse: review of reviews. Health Development Agency, London. www.hda-online.org.uk/documents/AlcoholSumPO.pdf

25  Kaner EF, Healther N, Brodie J *et al.* (2001) Patient and practitioner characteristics predict brief alcohol intervention in primary care. *British Journal of General Practice.* **471**: 822–7.

26  Anderson P (1993) Effectiveness of general practice interventions for patients with harmful alcohol consumption. *British Journal of General Practice.* **43**: 386–9.

27  Aira M, Kauhanen J, Larivaara P and Rautio P (2003) Factors influencing inquiry about patients' alcohol consumption by primary health care physicians: qualitative semi-structured interview study. *Family Practice.* **20**: 270–5.

28  World Health Organization (2000) Diagnosis and management of alcohol misuse in primary care. Reproduced in: G Foord-Kelcey (2003) *Guidelines.* **20**: 153–5.

29  Department of Health (1999) *Bulletin on Cervical Screening Programme: England 1998–9*. Department of Health, London. Also available from www.cancerscreening.nhs.uk/cervical

30  National Institute for Clinical Excellence. Guidance on the use of liquid-based cytology for cervical screening. www.nice.org.uk/pdf/TA69_LBC_review_FullGuidance.pdf

31  Sasieni P, Adams J and Cusik J (2003) Benefits of cervical screening at different ages: evidence from the UK audit of screening histories. *British Journal of Cancer.* **89(1)**: 88–93.

32  Department of Health (2003) *Job Evaluation Handbook*. Version 1. Department of Health, London.

# 5

# Contraception

**Case study 5.1**

Tracey is 16 years old. She comes to see you with her friend, Sharon, and asks if she can go on the pill. She tells you that she doesn't want to see her GP because he is a friend of the family and she thinks he would tell her mother.

# What issues you should cover

## Contraceptive care and confidentiality

Tell Tracey that health professionals are bound by a code of confidentiality. This means that they should not inform anyone other than a person who needs to know in order to help with medical care. No one else needs to know unless there is a risk to Tracey's health or to someone else's health, which would mean that other people would need to know. Ensure she knows that it would always be discussed with her if confidential information needed to be passed to someone else. You would like to let her GP know about the contraceptive consultation but only if she agrees. Give her the choice of being seen by herself or with her friend. Do not assume that, because she is with her friend, she wants to be seen with her friend. There may be peer pressure to accompany her, but this may restrict the information that she is willing to disclose (e.g. if she has had a termination of pregnancy that the friend doesn't know about).

## Risk of pregnancy

Explain that you need to know a bit about her to find out if it is safe for her to start taking the contraceptive pill. First, establish if she is already sexually active. If she is, then you need to know if she is using any other method of contraception (e.g. condoms). Ask if, and when, she has had any unprotected sexual intercourse and the date of her last menstrual period, in case she needs emergency contraception or is already pregnant (see information on emergency contraception later in this chapter).

If she has not started having sexual intercourse, explain that although lots of young people pretend to be having sexual intercourse, confidential surveys have shown that eight out of ten young people under the age of 16 years have not actually started having sexual intercourse. It may be better for her to go on the pill just in case but she does not have to have sexual intercourse unless she wants to.

## Age and the law

You may not be given correct information about her date of birth (or her identity) if she is fearful that she will not be given contraceptive advice because she is under 16 years of age. If she is living in the parental home, whatever her age, it is much simpler for her to have discussed her need for contraception at home so that there is no need for concealment of her attendance for advice or contraceptive supplies. Discuss how she might do this, if she has not already done so. The younger the woman, the more important it is to establish whether this discussion has taken place and whether the woman herself understands the full implications of her actions. Keep in mind the Fraser guidelines (*see* Chapter 3).

## Her plans for the future

Find out if Tracey is aware of other methods of contraception or whether she has simply opted for the pill because she only knows about the pill. Enquire about what type of relationship she is in now, how long she has been with this partner and if this is her only partner. Ensure that you do this sensitively and in a matter-of-fact way, so that you do not appear 'nosey' or intrusive. Tell her that you want to make sure that she is not being persuaded into sexual activity she does not want. Explain that you also need to know whether she needs protection from sexually transmitted infections (with condoms) as well as pregnancy. If the reasons behind your questions are clear, Tracey may be more inclined to answer in a full and non-threatened way. It is important not to appear judgemental and not to allow your personal values to interfere with the consultation. For example, if Tracey admits to having multiple sexual partners this should be accepted as a fact. Just ensure that Tracey is aware of the potential health risks associated with her behaviour (e.g. increased risk of sexually transmitted infections). If she says that she feels pressurised to have sexual intercourse, discuss how she could be more assertive (without putting herself at risk of violence). If Tracey says that she is not bothered whether she gets pregnant or not, this may be because she has no belief in her own ability to control her future – or because she does not have any vision of her future at all; things just happen to her. Talking to her about what she wants to do in the future can help her to see when a pregnancy might be more easily managed.

It may be extremely important for her not to become pregnant. Women who have definite plans – for a job, for training or further education – are usually well motivated to use contraception. Some young women are definite (at least for the time being) that they never want children.

## Reasons why she may not have used contraception

The Social Exclusion Unit report attributes high rates of teenage conception in the UK to young people's:[1]

* low expectations
* lack of knowledge about contraception and how it can be obtained

- lack of understanding about what is involved in forming relationships and parenting
- reception of mixed messages from society – 'it sometimes seems as if sex is compulsory but contraception is illegal' as one of the young people cited in the report said.

In a national survey of 515 teenagers aged 12 to 17 years, more than half of the respondents said that the main reason young people do not use birth control was because of drinking alcohol or using drugs. Boys and girls gave similar answers. Half of the teenagers quizzed thought another common reason for young people having unprotected sex was pressure from partners who do not want to use contraception. Young adolescents aged 12 to 14 years were as likely as the older teenagers to say this.[2]

## Problems associated with teenage pregnancy

The death rate for babies of teenage mothers is 60% higher than that for babies of older mothers. Maternal and foetal risks are highest in under-16 year olds.

Pregnant teenagers are more likely than mothers aged 20 to 35 years to have low income, poor education, be unwed, be cigarette smokers, and have poor nutrition. The Acheson report on health inequalities recognised that teenage mothers and children are at higher risk of experiencing adverse health, educational, social and economic outcomes, compared to older mothers and their children.[3]

Teenage pregnancy is a cause and effect of inequalities in health. Teenage mothers tend to have poor antenatal care, low birth weight infants and higher infant mortality rates. Teenage parents tend to miss out on education and have substantially lower incomes. They are more likely to suffer from postnatal depression and relationship breakdown. Risk factors for teenage pregnancy include: having a teenage mother, divorced parents, deprivation, being a child living in care, educational problems, sexual abuse, ethnicity, mental health problems and crime.[2]

## What she may know about contraception already

Some young women are well informed and have read many leaflets. Others know little or nothing. Make sure that you establish how much she already knows about the pill so that you can build on this knowledge and dismiss false beliefs. Using a leaflet that summarises all the methods enables you to go through each method and its level of contraceptive protection quite rapidly, so that she can make her own choice for discussion in more detail.[4]

## Check that she is safe to use her chosen contraceptive

Most young women will be healthy and have no contraindications to any method of contraception. For them, any method of contraception is preferable to the risks of pregnancy (although you can tell her that abstinence is the safest method of all, provided it does not fail!). You need to take a medical history to ensure that her chosen method will not do harm. Checking her blood pressure before giving contraceptives containing oestrogen is essential, but other physical examination is not necessary unless indicated by the history. Obesity and/or smoking increase her risks of venous thrombosis and cardiovascular disease. The absolute risk of venous thrombosis in a young woman is small, but lifestyle advice now may help her to make changes to avoid an increased risk in the future. However, keep in mind that she has come for contraceptive advice, not a lecture on her bad habits – or she will not want to return to see you.

You may wish to use a checklist to exclude contraindications. The World Health Organization (WHO) publishes a checklist with advice on cautions and contraindications.[5] A UK adaptation of the WHO advice appears on the website for the Faculty of Family Planning and Reproductive Health Care.[6]

## Summarising where the consultation has reached

The consultation has probably already lasted 10 minutes. You may need to summarise where you are and ask her what she wants to do next. If she has an urgent need for contraception (most young people do not attend until they do need it urgently) your next action is to take the extra time to help her learn how to use the method she has chosen. If she wants to use a long-acting method, she might be better using a short-acting method temporarily and returning later. This gives both of you time to discuss the method in more depth and for a more considered decision on a method that she cannot change easily. (Long-acting methods are discussed later in this chapter in Table 5.1.)

She and her sexual partner should use condoms for protection against method failure (common when people first start using contraception) and against sexually transmitted infections (STIs). She should be clear that most people do not have any symptoms from STIs and that appearances are no guide as to whether someone is infected or not.

A young woman who is still living with her parents or guardians can be helped to realise that they may be worried about whether she is protected against pregnancy, but may be uncertain how to ask her if she is at risk. Talk about ways she might discuss this with them.

## Using short-acting methods

### Condoms

You may be working in a situation where you are able to supply condoms but, if not, you need to know how she can obtain them. If you supply them, show her how they are used and give her a leaflet for her partner. Discuss with her how she is going to ask her partner to use condoms, how she will carry them (many young people do not have handbags or pockets) and that the condom should be put on the penis after erection but before genital contact.

Make sure that she knows she can obtain free supplies from family planning clinics, sexual health clinics and youth clinics, such as Brook or locally developed services. You should know where the local suppliers are, when they are open, and how she can be seen (does she need an appointment or is it open access?). She can go with her sexual partner or he can obtain condoms from the same places himself, so that he can be sure how to use them correctly. She, or her partner, can buy condoms from many outlets, including vending machines, chemists, supermarkets and garages.

Female condoms (Femidom) need to be used carefully so that the penis is placed inside the polyurethane sleeve lining the vagina. They are rather expensive – but can be bought over the counter with no need for medical intervention. They are disliked by some people because of the 'plastic mac' feel, and are noisy in use.

## Oral methods

She may decide to start on the combined oral contraceptive (COC) or the progestogen only pill (POP). It is useful to go through the leaflet with her that you will give her to take away.[4] This ensures that the advice you give and the advice in the leaflet is the same (or that you have hand-written any changes and explained the reasons for them). Tell her that the leaflet in the packet of pills may give slightly different advice depending on how long ago it was written. It may also be worth mentioning that information included within the packet of pills must, by law, include all known side-effects – however rare – so that this information sheet can appear quite frightening. Putting the risks in context for her may help her to establish the degree of risk involved.

Give her the choice of starting immediately or waiting for the first day of her next period. If she starts immediately, she should not rely on the pill for her contraception for the first seven days. If she starts on the first day of her menstrual cycle, she will be protected against pregnancy from that day, but will still need to use condoms for extra safety and protection against the risk of STIs.

Help her to decide what time of day will be easiest for her to remember to take her pill. Show her a packet of the pill she will be taking or a diagram in the leaflet of how to take the pill. Show her the section in the leaflet on what to do if she misses a pill, and go through the instructions, as this is the commonest cause of failure. Advise her how to stop smoking if she is a cigarette smoker.

Ask her to contact you (explain how) or attend again before her review appointment if she has any queries that are not explained in the leaflet, or new serious health complaints. Point out the types of condition, listed in the leaflet, that should make her return urgently (e.g. shortness of breath, leg pain and swelling, first or worsening migraine, or dizziness).

## Emergency contraception[7-9]

One of the reasons Tracey may be consulting you urgently rather than her own GP could be that she has had unprotected sexual intercourse and requires emergency contraception. The oral emergency contraceptives Levonelle or Levonelle-2 can be used up to 72 hours after unprotected intercourse, but the earlier the better. Levonelle and Levonelle-2 both contain the same doses of progestogen. Levonelle is the version bought over the counter and Levonelle-2 is the prescribed version. Levonelle is 95% effective in preventing pregnancy when taken within 24 hours of unprotected sexual intercourse. It is 85% effective when taken 25–48 hours later and only 58% effective when taken between 49 and 72 hours later.

Increased doses of hormone are necessary for patients on hepatic enzyme inducers such as phenytoin, carbamezepine or rifampicin to obtain the same blood levels. Most guidelines advise two pills followed by either another one or two 12 hours later.[7] Box 5.1 summarises the information you will need to elicit to decide whether oral emergency contraception should be prescribed and what advice to give. You could use this within a patient group direction to enable nurses in your organisation to administer Levonelle without a doctor having to sign for it. Department of Health guidelines on drawing up patient group directions (PGDs) are explicit, and ensure that, if adhered to, nurses administering drugs (such as Levonelle) without a doctor's involvement have medico-legal protection.[10] The use of patient group directions in circumstances such as giving emergency contraception can enable more patients to receive treatment promptly, maximising effectiveness.

---

**Box 5.1:**    Emergency contraception tablets – basic information required and advice

**Minimum information** to be recorded in the notes prior to prescribing oral postcoital contraception should include:

- last menstrual period (LMP)
- cycle length
- date and time of unprotected sexual intercourse (UPSI)
- day of cycle of UPSI
- any other UPSI since LMP
- options discussed (oral/IUD)
- any interacting medication
- current liver disease.

**Counselling** should include explaining:

- likelihood of nausea
- mode of action
- failure rate
- side-effects
- timing of next period
- action to take if next period is not on time
- discussion of future contraception needs.

**Vomiting after taking emergency combined oral contraception**
- If the patient vomits within two hours of taking the pills, she should be advised to seek further medical advice. Domperidone 10 mg can be used to prevent vomiting.

**Issuing guidelines**
- Negotiate the time the medication is to be taken and write it down.
- Go through the leaflet with the patient.
- Make follow-up arrangements or advise them to return one week after the expected date of the next period.
- Record whether emergency contraception was given or prescribed.

---

PGDs should be drawn up in accordance with the national guidance for England, Wales and Scotland and include:[10–12]

- the name of the organisation to which it applies
- the date it comes into effect and the date it expires
- a description of the contraceptive to which the PGD applies
- the type of health professional who may use the PGD (e.g. their qualifications or training required)
- the signature of the senior doctor or pharmacist and the representative of the health organisation involved
- a description of the circumstances in which the contraceptive can be used and those patients in whom it should not be used
- a description of the circumstances and arrangements for referral when appropriate
- details of how the contraceptive should be used and in what quantity and form it can be issued
- any warnings and side-effects
- what follow-up arrangements are to be made
- the nature of the record for audit purposes.

Both the nurse who will use the PGD, and the doctor authorising that the PGD can be used, should sign the PGD. The nurse and the doctor need to be satisfied that the nurse is competent to carry out the PGD.

Nurses who have qualified as extended and supplementary prescribers are able to independently prescribe most contraceptive pills (including Levonelle) if this falls within their scope of practice. More information on the range of drugs that can be prescribed by nurses can be found on the Department of Health website.[13]

The insertion of a copper IUD up to five days after unprotected intercourse has an even lower failure rate (0.1%) than oral methods. It can be used up to five days after the calculated date of ovulation (i.e. the 19th day of a 28-day shortest cycle from the history, counting day 1 as the first day of bleeding) and successfully prevents implantation. The IUD can be removed at the next menstruation if it is not required or desired for continuing contraception.

Remember that exposure to unprotected intercourse means exposure to possible sexual infection also, so informed consent for screening, especially for chlamydial infection, is usually required.

## Long-acting contraception

Tracey may wish to discuss her options if she wants to embark on long-acting contraception. If you have not got enough time to go through the alternatives in full detail you may supply her with leaflets or an audiotape about the possible types shown in Table 5.1 and arrange to see her again soon. Remember to exclude pregnancy with a pregnancy test if necessary before starting her on a long-acting method. Provide the contraception at the right time of her menstrual cycle, for example, you would give Depo-Provera, or insert an implant, within the first five days after her period has started.

**Table 5.1:**   Longer-acting methods of contraception

| Method | For | Against |
| --- | --- | --- |
| **Injection**<br>Depo-Provera: medroxy-progesterone acetate 150 mg given intramuscularly every 12 weeks, or Noristerat: norethisterone oenanthate 200 mg every 8 weeks | Could be started with the next period or before if pregnancy can be excluded. Effective after seven days, possibly sooner.<br>Lasts for 12 weeks (or 8 weeks for Noristerat), giving time to consider longer-term action.<br>Usually gives very light and infrequent periods or no bleeding at all.<br>Enhances breast milk flow. Is likely to give very light or absent menses once breast feeding has stopped.<br>Very low failure rate. | Weight gain common with Depo-Provera, less with Noristerat. The patient has to return every 12 (or 8) weeks for another injection and may easily forget unless someone else takes the responsibility for reminding her. Progestogenic side-effects may be unacceptable: acne, feeling constantly premenstrual, irregular or absent periods.<br>She may not have attained her peak bone mass because of her age, especially if she smokes or has a poor diet. Depo-Provera might increase the risk of a low bone mass.<br>Small theoretical risk to a breast-fed baby from the absorbed progestogen, especially if a baby is premature and has immature liver enzymes. |
| **Implant**<br>Implanon: small plastic rod inserted in the bicipital groove of the upper arm releasing etonorgestrel over three years | She would not require any other method for three years, giving time for reflection about her future needs.<br>If someone in the practice or clinic fits implants, she could have one fitted within five days of the start of her next period.<br>She does not have to remember anything for three years.<br>Very low failure rate. | Usually cannot be done immediately and needs some time to set up a fitting.<br>If no one in the practice or clinic fits these, the patient may have to attend another venue. Frequent spotting or light periods may not suit everyone and a few people have unacceptable progestogenic side-effects.<br>Recall system needed so that the implant is not forgotten. |
| **Intrauterine device with copper (IUCD)**<br>e.g. T-safe CU 380A, Multiload Cu 375, Nova-T 380, Flexi-T 300, Gynefix | Could be fitted immediately if facilities are available and pregnancy can be excluded. | Might have to re-attend or attend a different venue if no facilities are available to fit it immediately. Easier to fit in the multiparous uterus. |

**Table 5.1:**   Continued

| Method | For | Against |
| --- | --- | --- |
| | Would give protection between five and ten years depending on device. T-safe CU 380A has a very low failure rate with the others only slightly higher. Can be used as a post-coital method if she is at risk following unprotected intercourse. | Success rates are dependent more on the expertise of the person fitting it than on the type of device used. Health professionals who only fit a few devices each year have higher expulsion, bleeding, removal and perforation rates. Usually increases the menstrual loss and may increase dysmenorrhoea if present. Recall system needed so that it is not forgotten. |
| **Intrauterine system with progesterone (IUS)** Mirena | Could be fitted within five days of the start of her next period if facilities are available. Decreases menstrual loss, usually to none after the first few months of irregular loss. Would give protection for five years. Failure rate is even lower than for sterilisation. | Might have to re-attend or attend a different venue if no facilities are available to fit it immediately. Nulliparous women usually need cervical anaesthesia, as the diameter of the device is wider than an IUD. Success rates are dependent more on the expertise of the person fitting it than on the type of device used. Specific training is needed as it has a different insertion technique from other IUCDs. Decreases menstrual loss, usually to none after the first few months of irregular loss. Recall system needed so that it is not forgotten. |
| **Female sterilisation** | Permanent and suitable for women who are certain they want no more children. Low failure rate. | Permanent and not suitable for anyone who is not certain or feels they will have lost their femininity. Failure rate higher than vasectomy or IUS. Usually requires referral to secondary care (long wait to be seen) and at least admission for day case surgery. Usually done under general anaesthesia with the attendant risks. |

**Table 5.1:**   Continued

| Method | For | Against |
|---|---|---|
| | | May require laparotomy if the tubes cannot be visualised with the laparoscope. That would require a longer stay in hospital and longer recovery period. |
| **Vasectomy** | Permanent and suitable for men who are certain they want no more children. Low failure rate. | Not suitable for anyone who is not certain about whether more children will ever be desired. Usually done under local anaesthesia, occasionally under general with its attendant risks. Temporary pain and discomfort in most men who can return to work after 48 hours. Manual workers require longer off work. Some men develop epididymal cysts, or granulomas. Chronic pain develops in about 2% of men. |
| **Combined contraceptive patch** | Only needs application weekly for three weeks, omitted for the fourth week. Good cycle control. Under the control of the woman if she wants to stop it at any time. Low failure rate but not as low as any of the methods above. | The oestrogen component can reduce breast milk flow. The oestrogen component increases her thrombosis risk. She has to remember it weekly. It is expensive compared with the oral contraceptive pill. |

# Collecting data to demonstrate your learning, competence, performance and standards of service delivery

## Example of cycle of evidence 5.1

- Focus: clinical care
- Other relevant foci: probity, relationships with patients, relationships with colleagues

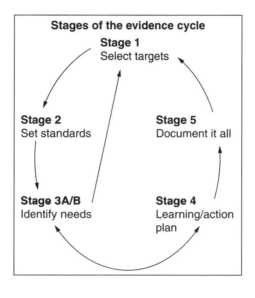

**Stages of the evidence cycle**

**Stage 1**
Select targets

**Stage 2**
Set standards

**Stage 5**
Document it all

**Stage 3A/B**
Identify needs

**Stage 4**
Learning/action plan

---

**Case study 5.2**

A new nurse is working alongside you as a locum practice nurse, while the regular practice nurse is on holiday. The new nurse appears very confident. At the end of the morning she asks if you would obtain a repeat prescription from the GP for emergency contraceptive pills that she supplied to a patient she saw earlier. On questioning, she tells you that she saw a 15-year-old girl who presented asking for the emergency pill. The patient told the nurse that it stated in the practice leaflet that practice nurses are able to provide patients with emergency contraception. The nurse confirmed this from the practice leaflet.

Because the locum nurse is not named within the PGD to administer Levonelle, you inform her that she should have referred the patient to you or a doctor. She tells you that you are over-reacting and that she is quite capable of giving out pills. She assures you that she checked the patient's blood pressure (which was normal) and ensured that unprotected sexual intercourse had occurred within the past 72 hours.

It is the responsibility of the employer (who, in this case, is likely to be the GP) to assess the competency of the locum nurse. However, if you, as senior nurse, are aware that she has not been named within a PGD then you are correct to point out that she was acting outside her limitations. This case should be discussed with the GP, locum nurse and yourself to ensure that the patient has not received inferior care. The patient may need to be contacted to ascertain whether all requirements within the PGD were met. As the patient in question is under 16 years, it is important to ensure that the Fraser guidelines have been applied, and that this is adequately documented.

This is just an example. Keep your task simple. You could choose three or four cycles of evidence to demonstrate your competence each year.

## Stage 1: Select your aspirations for good practice

The excellent nurse:

- responds rapidly to anomalies in clinical practice
- is supportive and approachable to colleagues
- arranges appropriate training for practice staff in collaboration with medical staff.

## Stage 2: Set the standards for your outcomes

> Outcomes might include:
>
> - the way learning is applied
> - a learnt skill
> - a protocol
> - a strategy that is implemented
> - meeting recommended standards.

- Demonstrate consistent best practice in provision of emergency contraception to teenagers in respect of availability and accessibility and clinical management.
- Demonstrate best practice in consistency of care from the entire healthcare team.
- Information about contraceptive services you provide, e.g. in the practice leaflet, is factual and verifiable, and conforms with the law and guidance issued by the Advertising Standards Agency.
- Information published about your services does not exploit patients' vulnerability or lack of medical knowledge, or put pressure on staff to deliver a service where this is outside their normal remit.

## Stage 3A: Identify your learning needs

- Carry out with other practice staff a review of the expected role of locum staff and clarify the role and responsibility of other nurses who work with them.
- Identify what role you might have in assessing the competency of locum staff – you may wish to contact the clinical governance lead within the PCT to determine whether there are standards in place for locum practice nurses, and what part you might play in their CPD.
- Review PGDs used within the workplace and ascertain whether these are for named nurses or for 'all nurses working within the organisation'. Consider if it is helpful and safe to include all nurses.

## Stage 3B: Identify your service needs

> Any of the needs assessment exercises in 3A may also reveal service needs.

- Audit the need for nurse-led family planning services, which may involve the use of PGDs e.g. a patient survey to establish the interval between the time an appointment is requested for a repeat prescription of the contraceptive pill and the time the prescription is issued.
- Determine how competency of locum nursing staff is assessed and documented e.g. you may wish to designate assessment of basic competency in specialist areas

(such as sexual health) to nurses who are known to have a special interest or a high level of proficiency. Locum nurses may need to have competencies signed off before being able to work without direct supervision.

- Check with staff that everyone is aware of the training needs required before the use of PGDs and ensure that training is readily available as required.
- Ask the PCO or other external commentators to critique the information you supply about your contraceptive services (practice leaflet or other published information).

## Stage 4: Make and carry out a learning and action plan

- Read up on the latest recommendations for emergency contraception[7] and revise the PGD if required.
- Read up and discuss at a practice meeting the latest evidence about progestogen-only emergency contraception.[14,15]
- Visit other practices to discuss how excellent and appropriate care for teenagers and/or family planning services is maintained or managed in alternative ways during staff shortages.
- Rewrite the sections in the practice leaflet relating to the provision of nursing services. Ensure these are informative and accurate and that all nurses have had an opportunity to comment on them before the leaflet is sent for printing.
- Analyse your reactions to the events in your reflective diary.

## Stage 5: Document your learning, competence, performance and standards of service delivery

- Re-audit and record the consistent application of PGDs relating to emergency contraception.
- Record the teenage patient survey for timely access and the actions taken.
- Record the events, suitably anonymised, from your reflective diary together with your analysis of your reactions and the changes that you initiated. Show how you learnt from difficult experiences and improved the safety of your practice.
- Record the discussion with staff relating to the limitation of locum nursing services.
- Ensure that the practice leaflet describing nursing services provided in the practice is written and reviewed by nurses.

---

**Case study 5.2 continued**

After a joint discussion between yourself, the locum nurse and the GP, you found that there is inadequate information recorded and uncertainty about the advice given. The GP felt it would be too threatening if he contacted the patient and you and the locum nurse agreed. You offered to contact the school nurse who arranged to speak to the girl later that day.

The school nurse established that Levonelle had been taken and that un-protected sexual intercourse had occurred on day 21 of a 28-day cycle. She warned the patient that her period could arrive earlier or later than usual (or on time!). She advised the girl to visit the practice nurse again in two weeks' time (so that a pregnancy test can be done if she has not had a period and that future contraception can be discussed). The school nurse also agreed to call into the surgery and document her findings and adherence to Fraser guidelines in the medical notes.

You use this event as an opportunity to educate the locum nurse about emergency contraception. She is advised not to administer any drugs without first checking the procedure with another nurse or doctor in the practice. The locum nurse confesses that she did not realise there were so many interesting things to learn about contraceptive care and resolves to undertake the family planning training course.

# Example cycle of evidence 5.2

- Focus: clinical care
- Other relevant foci: relationships with patients, keeping up to date, extending your role, working with colleagues

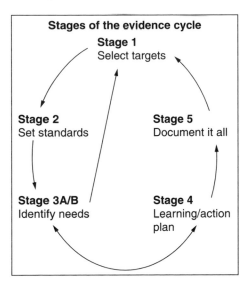

**Stages of the evidence cycle**

**Stage 1**
Select targets

**Stage 2**
Set standards

**Stage 5**
Document it all

**Stage 3A/B**
Identify needs

**Stage 4**
Learning/action plan

**Case study 5.3**

Mrs Daffy tells you that her husband says she must be sterilised. She delivered her fifth child six weeks ago and has had two miscarriages as well. She has been prescribed some progestogen-only pills to start on the 21st day after delivery but says she has not had time to obtain them from the pharmacy yet. She adds that she doesn't like taking pills anyway. She is obviously overweight and from her medical record it can be seen that she is 29 years old and smokes but has a normal blood pressure. She asks if it is okay to breast feed the baby who is crying loudly and two of her other children start investigating the drawers and cupboards in the consulting room.

This is just an example. Keep your task simple. You could choose three or four cycles of evidence to demonstrate your competence each year.

## Stage 1: Select your aspirations for good practice

The excellent nurse:

- makes an adequate assessment of the patient's condition, based on the history and, if indicated, an appropriate examination
- provides or requests investigations or treatment where necessary
- recognises and works within the limits of his/her competence and refers to another practitioner when indicated
- seeks to empower and educate patients.

## Stage 2: Set the standards for your outcomes

Outcomes might include:

- the way learning is applied
- a learnt skill
- a protocol
- a strategy that is implemented
- meeting recommended standards.

- Demonstrate consistent best practice in provision of continuing contraception to patients in respect of availability and accessibility and clinical management.
- The best use of resources is demonstrated.
- You can show how you contribute to patient education.
- You can show how you act as patients' advocate.

## Stage 3A: Identify your learning needs

- Carry out a significant event audit with other practice staff e.g. looking at the reasons why Mrs Daffy, or a similar patient, had not used contraception previously. Had she defaulted from care or had there been failures in the system or standards of care?
- Examine a complaint e.g. about inadequate counselling before sterilisation or vasectomy. Do you need to use an up-to-date leaflet or a checklist to ensure that people have sufficient information to make an informed choice?
- Keep a reflective diary capturing trends or comments relating to problems or issues of longer-acting methods of contraception e.g. you might record that you feel less confident in talking about sterilisation because it is a procedure in which you are not personally involved.

## Stage 3B: Identify your service needs

Any of the needs assessment exercises in 3A may also reveal service needs.

- Review the difficulty of arranging for an IUD, IUS or implant to be fitted promptly because of appointment difficulties or availability of an adequately qualified doctor who can fit such devices.
- Perform a patient survey to ascertain the demand and when people would like to be able to access a service providing longer-acting methods.
- Audit the availability and adequacy of emergency resuscitation equipment and the training standards of health professionals to use it.
- Review the services available to care for children during personal consultations where parents would welcome privacy.

## Stage 4: Make and carry out a learning and action plan

- Find out if there is demand, and training available, for nurses to learn how to fit and remove IUDs, IUSs and implants.
- Research the availability of provision of longer-acting methods of contraception and liaise with those services. Perhaps you might help to make a proposal to the PCO for more accessible local provision. This might involve finding out the comparative costs of various contraceptive options and promoting the cause of nurse-led training to initiate or fit long-term methods.

- Read up about alternative methods of contraception and the points to consider about sterilisation counselling.
- Contact the health visitor to discuss the family circumstances and identify who is most appropriate and best qualified to work with this patient regarding her contraceptive choices at the current time.

### Stage 5: Document your learning, competence, performance and standards of service delivery

- Retain any certificates of learning and competence achieved.
- Record and disseminate your learning about other contraceptive provision.
- Record referrals you have made to other healthcare professionals in your reflective diary.
- Record the outcome of the significant event audit.
- Record the results of the patient survey of their needs and preferences for services for obtaining long-acting methods of contraception, and any representations made to the PCO.
- Record the conclusions from your discussion with the health visitor about the best provision of advice for this patient.

---

**Case study 5.3 continued**

It was clearly impossible to undertake an adequate assessment initially. You liaised with the health visitor who agreed to call and discuss contraceptive options with Mrs Daffy. The health visitor also impressed on Mrs Daffy the need to initiate childcare when discussing such important issues as sterilisation in order to have adequate thinking time.

Mrs Daffy refused the offer of an immediate injection or pill. She was able to get her sister to look after the older children, while she just brought the baby to the surgery. One of the receptionists was able to look after the baby after he had been fed and was in his pushchair. You are able to have a full discussion of the options for contraception. She says her husband would never 'be done'. She decides she definitely wants an IUS after all the advantages and disadvantages are explained. You manage to arrange an IUS fitting for the following week.

---

# References

1 Department of Health (1999) *Teenage Pregnancy*. Social Exclusion Unit, Department of Health, London.

2 Chambers R, Wakley G and Chambers S (2001) *Tackling Teenage Pregnancy: sex culture and needs*. Radcliffe Medical Press, Oxford.

3 Acheson D (chair) (1998). *Independent Inquiry into Inequalities in Health Report*. The Stationery Office, London.

4 The general leaflet 'Contraception', those on individual methods, and a good range of other leaflets, are available from FPA, 2–12 Pentonville Road, London N1 9FP, tel: 020 7837 5432.

5 World Health Organization (2000) *Improving Access to Quality Care in Family Planning*. WHO, Geneva. www.who.int/reproductive-health

6 www.ffprhc.org.uk/

7 Faculty of Family Planning and Reproductive Health Care: Clinical Effectiveness Unit (2003) FFPRHC Guidance: emergency contraception. *British Journal of Family Planning and Reproductive Health Care*. **29(2)**: 9–16 and www.ffprhc.org.uk (publications).

8 Wakley G and Chambers R (2002) *Sexual Health Matters in Primary Care*. Radcliffe Medical Press, Oxford.

9 Belfield T (1999) *Contraceptive Handbook* (3e). Family Planning Association, London.

10 Department of Health (2000) *Health Service Circular 2000/026 Patient Group Directions*. Department of Health, London.

11 The National Welsh Assembly (2000) *Review of Prescribing, Supply and Administration of Medicines by Health Professionals under Patient Group Directions (PGD)*. The Welsh Assembly, Cardiff.

12 Scottish Executive Health Department NHS (2001) *Patient Group Directions*. www.show.scot.nhs.uk/sehd/mels/HDL2001_07.htm

13 www.dh.gov.uk and enter 'nurse prescribing' into the search box to obtain the most recent information.

14 Ellertson C, Evans M, Ferden S *et al.* (2003) Extending the time limit for starting the Yupze regimen of emergency contraception to 120 hours. *Obstetrics and Gynecology*. **101(6)**: 1168–71.

15 von Hertzen H, Piaggio G, Ding J *et al.* (2002) Low dose mifepristone and two regimens of levonorgestrel for emergency contraception: a WHO multicentre randomised trial. *Lancet*. **360(9348)**: 1803–10.

# Further reading

- Belfield T (1999) *Contraceptive Handbook* (3e). Family Planning Association, London.
- Guillebaud J (1999) *Contraception: your questions answered*. Churchill Livingstone, London.
- Rowlands S (1997) *Managing Family Planning in General Practice*. Radcliffe Medical Press, Oxford.
- Royal College of Obstetricians and Gynaecologists (1998) *Male and Female Sterilisation*. Royal College of Obstetricians and Gynaecologists, London.
- Wakley G and Chambers R (2002) *Sexual Health Matters in Primary Care*. Radcliffe Medical Press, Oxford.
- Wakley G, Cunnion M and Chambers R (2003) *Improving Sexual Health Advice*. Radcliffe Medical Press, Oxford.

# 6

## Sexually transmitted infections

---

**Case study 6.1**

A 21-year-old woman attends a nurse-led sexual health clinic telling you that her recent ex-partner has sent her a text message accusing her of giving him an infection. She has little other information except that he has been to the genitourinary medicine (GUM) clinic in the next town. She refuses to attend the GUM clinic and wants you to treat her.

---

# What issues you should cover[1]

## Giving information about genitourinary (GUM) clinics

Access to GUM clinics varies across the country and new users often find it difficult to know what is available. People are often fearful of attending because of perceived stigma, or just because going somewhere new always provokes anxiety – and it is difficult to ask a friend to go with them for support. You should know where the clinics are and how people can be seen. It is a good idea to visit the clinic yourself – this will enable you to give more detail to patients (e.g. where the nearest car park is, or what the reception area is like). Passing on this sort of detailed information can help to reduce patients' anxiety. It may mean that they are more inclined to visit the clinic because they feel less fearful about what they can expect. Some clinics have open access while others require appointments to be made by telephone. Some are open in the evening, others from 10am to 5pm (not very convenient!). Some of the clinics now have a seamless one-stop service together with contraceptive clinics or are on the same premises to allow for easy transfers between services.

Stress that the service is confidential and that the records are kept separately from other hospital records. By law, staff in a GUM clinic cannot tell a patient if or what STI their partner has, or tell their doctor that they have attended unless the patient requests it. The clinic cannot give any information to other doctors, solicitors, insurance companies or the police without the consent of the patient. The clinic will record a name and a date of birth, and will ask for a contact address so that results can be given (but patients do not have to give this information if they prefer not to).

After a detailed history, often using a checklist, tests can be done immediately to diagnose some infections. Other tests will take some time for the results to be known. The clinic does need some identifying information so that they can access patients' records when they re-attend. All treatment is free of charge and this can be a potent incentive to attend if treatment is needed. Reimbursement of travel expenses can also sometimes be made.

The patient needs to be clear that you will not be able to give such a complete service in most sexual health clinics in the community partly because of limitations for carrying out testing. However, the Sexual Health Strategy stresses that more clinics should emerge to provide both routine sexual health advice and facilities for treatment for infections within one centre.[2] Results of testing are more reliable if the patient travels to the hospital laboratory with her samples still in her in the body than if you take samples and transport them separately. For many tests, the pick up rate from samples falls the longer the delay between testing and examination of the specimens.

# Taking a sexual history[1]

If she still refuses to attend the GUM clinic, then you must do your best for her. Explain the reason for taking a sexual history. If patients understand why questions are being asked they will be more likely to talk fully and less likely to be offended or misinterpret your intentions. Ask the patient if it is all right to carry on.

Make sure the patient knows that you are bound by confidentiality, and under what circumstances you would need to pass information on – mention this early on and explain how the information given will be kept confidential and who will have access to that information.

Consider asking their partner to participate or to supply information if the patient agrees (unlikely in this case). If a partner does attend, encourage one-to-one discussion, as some issues involve sexual activity with other partners or information that one of a couple would not want the other to hear.

Listen carefully – allow the patient to guide the discussion and introduce the terminology. This does not imply that you should use the same language or slang as patients do. Using physiologically accurate terms, e.g. penis, vagina, will maintain a sense of professional distance that many patients find reassuring. Be careful to define the words that you and the patient use. The vagina or uterus mean something specific to you, but the terms may be used in a much wider sense by patients to indicate any part of the female genitals. Similarly, someone may talk about 'going to bed with someone' and you need to be clear whether this actually includes sexual penetration. 'Making love' may include sexual penetration, or may refer to caressing and other sexual stimulation. There are problems too with identifying the sex of the partner; 'Pat' or 'Lesley' could be either. Always check that what you understood is actually what the patient meant.

Ask the patient to tell you about her sexual activity. It may be necessary to direct some questions by giving examples, as some patients may be coy about volunteering information, but are happy to respond to direct questions e.g. have you had oral sex? Explain each time why you are asking those particular questions. Other forms of sexual activity should also be specified, depending on the patient's sexual orientation. You will need to explain that you need to know the areas of the body that might become infected (throat, rectum, etc) so that investigations are complete but relevant.

Ask about symptoms, but bear in mind (and tell the patient) that most people with an STI do not have any symptoms. Has she had any burning when she passes water, any change in her vaginal secretions, any soreness, rash or lumps in the genital area, or any irregular bleeding between periods or after intercourse? Has there been any change in the amount of her period loss or any episodes of abdominal pain?

Enquire about any previous STI and her own perception of her risk. An estimate can be made from the length of time she was with that partner and how many other sexual partners she has had in the last 12 months.

## Give information about STIs

You need to find out what she knows about STIs. She may be reluctant to have any investigations performed if she has no symptoms. You can give her some information about how often people are infected in her age group and about her risks – adjusted for her level of comprehension. Then she will be in a better position to make an informed choice.

## Statistics about STIs[3]

Cases of *Chlamydia trachomatis* identified have doubled in the last six years. In 2000, genital chlamydial infection was the commonest bacterial STI seen. Highest rates of diagnosis of *Chlamydia* are seen in young people, particularly women in the 16 to 19 year and 20 to 24 year age groups.

Genital warts (HPV) are the commonest viral STI and also the commonest STI overall. The rise in the number of cases of gonorrhoea (GC) has been largest in the youngest age groups – 16 to 19 years and 20 to 24 years of age. The majority of cases identified have been in men – largely because women rarely have symptoms.

Genital herpes first attack rates have risen slightly. The rise in the numbers of new cases of syphilis that recently occurred was mainly in men who have sex with men.

Human immunodeficiency virus (HIV) infection rates continue to rise. HIV infection is now identified more commonly in heterosexuals than in homosexual men. Infection rates are increasing, perhaps due to a relaxation of the vigilance of people who believed that they were at risk and used condoms after publicity campaigns, but have now become complacent about the risk, as it is no longer in the news. Health professionals have a key role in arresting this complacency by continually alerting patients to the risks of all sexually transmitted infections (including HIV) when they discuss contraception and opportunistically discussing sexual health in consultations where health promotion is highlighted.

Hepatitis B rates have slightly decreased but hepatitis C rates have increased, perhaps reflecting the effect of immunisation against hepatitis B.

Some other infections that occur elsewhere in the body such as streptococcus (which usually causes skin and throat infections), or gut bacteria like *E. coli*, can be spread by sexual activity. Molluscum contagiosum is a very common infection, especially in children but can also be spread through sexual activity. Some other more unusual STIs may be seen occasionally in people returning from other countries.

Although thrush and bacterial vaginosis are not classified as STIs, they are common causes of genital infection. Thrush (also known as candida, or candidiasis) is not usually passed on from a woman to a man by sexual intercourse. It is a very common cause of vaginal discharge, soreness and itching. Bacterial vaginosis is possibly even more frequently found in women complaining of vaginal discharge.

# Knowledge about the individual infections[4]

Ask her what she knows about the infections to find out what other information she might need. Listening to her will also give you a feel for the level of information she may require at this stage. Support whatever information you give by leaflets (or similar) to take away, as afterwards she will only recall a small percentage of what you say in the consultation. Try to amass a wide range of leaflets that are targeted at differing needs (e.g. teenagers, older people, the intellectual and the non-intellectual) so that you have extensive resources to draw on in order to satisfy individual patients' needs.

## Chlamydia

In under-26 year olds, *Chlamydia* has been identified in about 10–12% of people in pilot studies of population screening. Chlamydial infection is frequently asymptomatic but is a common cause of infertility and chronic pelvic infection. It can cause ectopic pregnancy and chronic pelvic pain. Ascending infection in men causes epididymitis but evidence of male infertility is limited. Maternal to infant transmission causes neonatal conjunctivitis and pneumonia. It may co-exist with other STIs and may help in the transmission and acquisition of HIV infection.

## Gonorrhoea

The incidence of this infection is increasing especially among 16–19 year olds. Infection can be asymptomatic in about 10% of men and 50% of women. Male symptoms of dysuria, discharge or epididymitis, or female symptoms of discharge, dysuria or abdominal pain should raise your suspicions.

## Non-specific urethritis or non-specific genital infection

It is common in young men and is defined as an infection, usually urethritis, not caused by gonorrhoea. Up to 40% of episodes of urethritis are in fact caused by *Chlamydia*, so she will need tests for this. *Mycoplasma genitalium* and *Ureaplasma urealyticum* are commonest amongst the other causative organisms. The diagnosis is mainly made by a combination of symptoms of urethritis and the presence of pus cells – more than 5 per high power field (×400) – on a slide made from a urethral swab. The male partner will have been told to get his partner(s) treated to prevent recurrence. Treatment is as for *Chlamydia*.

## Genital warts: human papilloma virus (HPV)

First ever presentation of genital warts has shown a significant rise in the 16–19-year-old age group. HPV infection is common amongst sexually active young people whether or not visible warts are present. Small plane warts may be visible on examination without any symptoms being present. Genital warts are usually spread sexually, so their presence should prompt a search for other STIs. Some HPVs (types 16, 18, 31, 33 and 35) – not usually the ones presenting as visible warts – are associated with the development of cervical cancer and yearly cervical screening for five years is normally suggested if wart virus is found. Determining the type of HPV present is still a research technique.

## Syphilis

Although many people know that syphilis is an STI, new cases of syphilis in the UK are uncommon and are mostly found by screening in pregnancy or on blood donation. The presence of a solitary ulcer or the rash of secondary syphilis may raise suspicions.

## Viral hepatitis

Several different virus types cause hepatitis, all of which can cause an acute illness with jaundice. Asymptomatic infections are common. Hepatitis B and D also cause chronic infection progressing to cirrhosis and liver failure. Hepatitis B is more infectious than HIV and can be spread by sexual intercourse as well as from contaminated blood. Hepatitis A can be caught sexually from a partner with an active infection.

## Human immunodeficiency disease (HIV)

The symptoms of an acute infection with HIV may resemble glandular fever, but most new infections do not show any symptoms. The development of antibodies after infection takes about two to six weeks, but can be later than this. Chronic infection may also be asymptomatic, but about one-third of patients have generalised persistently enlarged lymph nodes. Later in the course of the chronic infection, symptoms of night sweats, fevers, diarrhoea and weight loss occur. Frequent infections of mucous membranes or skin are often present. About 75% of HIV-positive people develop symptoms over a 9–10 year period without therapy.

## Trichomonas vaginalis

This organism with a flagella occurs in the urethra in both sexes but also in the vagina and paraurethral glands in women. In adults it is a sexually transmitted infection and is frequently associated with other STIs. (Babies can acquire the infection perinatally from an infected mother.) The commonest complaint in both men and women is of discharge, but 15–50% of infected men have no symptoms. Women also complain of itching, dysuria or a smelly discharge. Although the discharge is classically described as frothy yellow, it is often variable both in consistency and colour.

*Bacterial vaginosis*

Bacterial vaginosis (BV) may be even more common than 'thrush'. It was formerly called 'Gardnerella vaginosis' and is the overgrowth of predominately anaerobic bacteria that are normally present in only small numbers in the healthy vagina. They produce a fishy or ammonia smell in alkaline conditions so the condition may be worse after intercourse or just after a woman's periods have finished. It is not a sexually transmitted infection.

BV is causing increasing concern to health professionals because of:

- pelvic inflammatory disease
- endometritis
- post-operative cuff infection after a transabdominal hysterectomy (TAH) and vaginal hysterectomy
- post-abortal infection
- psychosexual problems (the smell!)
- obstetric factors: increase in late miscarriage rates, chorioendometritis, pre-term delivery
- as a possible co-factor in HIV transmission.

*Thrush*

Sometimes this fungal infection may be reported on cervical smears or swabs taken for other reasons when there are no symptoms. The first attack can be extremely uncomfortable with the swelling, itching, soreness and discharge causing considerable distress. Although often described as typically presenting with white 'cottage cheese'-like patches over bright red areas of the vulval or vaginal walls, this is more frequent in pregnancy. The appearance of the discharge may be very variable and the vulva may be fissured or red and shiny from frequent scratching. Most women complain mainly of:

- itching and soreness
- rapid onset often in the pre-menstrual week
- painful urination and/or sexual intercourse.

It is not classified as an STI infection and rarely spreads between partners.

# Investigations that may be needed

You need to discuss with the woman what tests you can do, how long the results will take and how she will obtain the results (*see* Table 6.1). She may be happy for you to contact her at home but, if not, other arrangements must be made such as sending them to a trusted friend. If she does not give consent to be contacted then it is essential that she understands that she must re-attend for the results.

**Table 6.1:** Suggested investigations for screening for an STI indicated by the history

| Test | Useful for |
| --- | --- |
| High vaginal swab (HVS) in Stuart's or similar transport medium | Candida and bacterial vaginosis (not STIs), trichomonas |
| Cervical exudate swab or endocervical swab and urethral swab in Stuart's or similar transport medium | Gram stain shows gram-negative diplococcus in about half of all gonococcal infections; culture as well will detect about 90% of infections |
| Chlamydia test: know which testing procedure your microbiology department uses. If it is enzyme immuno-assay (EIA) send an endocervical swab and urethral swab. Use the special chlamydial testing kit supplied by your laboratory for taking samples from the cervix. Follow the instructions that come with the pack from the laboratory as each type of pack has different instructions. Some are very clear and state that the cleaning swab (the large bulbous swab of the two) must not be used as the swab for Chlamydia. First clean any mucus off the cervix with the cleaning swab and then use the Chlamydia swab (the metal- or plastic-handled, thin flat-ended swab). Rotate it for a minimum of 30 s in the cervix. Take cells from the transitional zone (the junction between the outer cells of the cervix and the inner ones lining the cervical canal). Remove the swab from the vagina and place it in the container supplied in accordance with the instructions. | Chlamydia trachomatis |
| First catch urine (not mid-stream urine (MSU)) | Nucleic acid amplification tests for Chlamydia and gonorrhoea* |
| Viral swabs from any ulcers or sores | Herpes simplex, Candida |
| Swabs from other sites e.g. pharynx, rectum | Gonorrhoea |
| Blood test | Viral hepatitis or HIV |

*Nucleic acid amplification tests have been developed that are highly sensitive (over 90%) compared with the standard endocervical EIA test that has a lower sensitivity of 60% to 70%. These tests may also be called polymerisation chain reaction (PCR) tests. New combined gonorrhoea/Chlamydia PCR screening tests are available for urine testing. You will need to know what the standards are for your laboratory and their specificity rate (so that you know how many false positive and false negative results might be expected).

## Prevention of transmission[5]

It is important to ensure that any infection is not spread to any other partner(s). Partner notification is an important part of the control of STIs but is often difficult to achieve. The woman should be advised to abstain from intercourse until she has the results of screening and has been treated if necessary. Remember not all women are able to refuse to have sexual intercourse if there is an imbalance of power between the partners, or if cultural or religious customs prevent her expressing her wishes.

## Treatment[6,7]

If you can establish what infection her previous partner has been told he has, treatment for this infection could be started as soon as investigations are complete. She should only be treated empirically if you cannot obtain her consent to investigations. It is possible for her to have an infection that has not been identified in her previous partner. The reasons for this can be either he has not contracted an infection that she has, or because of the limitations of the test (that is, he has had a false negative test).

---

**Case study 6.1 continued**

Before she leaves the patient asks you why she was not screened for infections like *Chlamydia* when she had her recent cervical smear. You tell her some of what is described in Box 6.1 and the general principles of screening with special regard to *Chlamydia*.

---

# General principles to consider when introducing screening of well people for illnesses or infections

* *Is the condition important?* Chlamydia is an important cause of infertility, ectopic pregnancy, salpingitis, chronic pelvic pain and morbidity.
* *Is the natural history well understood?* Between 70% and 80% of women with cervical infections have no symptoms, but it is not clear how many have a risk of ascending infections in the absence of precipitating factors such as instrumentation of the uterus.
* *Is there a recognisable early stage?* Screening tests can identify infection when no symptoms are present.
* *Is there a suitable test?* The nucleic acid amplification tests are more sensitive and specific than the previous EIA tests and can be done on urine as well as swabs. Blood tests are not useful as they tell you only if someone has ever had the infection (and possibly got rid of it), not whether they have it currently.
* *Is the test acceptable?* Urine tests are more acceptable than cervical or urethral swabs. Self-taken swabs have also been shown to be useful and acceptable in some groups.
* *At what intervals should the test be repeated?* Unknown – and may depend on the accuracy and completeness of contact tracing and treatment, and on social factors like change of sexual partner or monogamy.
* *Are there adequate facilities for the diagnosis and treatment?* No: primary care health professionals do not always have sufficient time, skills or facilities for investigation, GUM clinics need increased resources to cope with the number of referrals of people with positive tests, the laboratories have insufficient capacity and resources to carry out the tests. Instigating a campaign about *Chlamydia* screening without increasing the facilities for screening, further testing for confirmation

and for treatment, would cause collapse of the present already overstretched arrangements.

- *Is treatment at an early stage of more benefit than treatment at a later stage?* Definitely: infection can easily be eradicated in the early stages before structural damage occurs. However, it is unknown how often people recover from chlamydial infection without treatment.
- *Are the chances of physical and psychological harm less than the chances of benefit?* This depends on how the test is presented, people's feelings about stigmatisation (having a 'sexually transmitted infection') and public knowledge about the condition.
- *Can the cost be balanced against the benefits the service provides, versus other opportunity costs and benefits?* Unknown as yet: pilot studies from Merseyside and Southampton showed much higher prevalence of infection and higher costs for the counselling time and number of tests performed than expected.[8,9]

You can read about setting up your own guidelines that might be part of a development plan in your workplace in the book *Sexual Health Matters in Primary Care*.[1]

## Managing infection control in primary care settings

You clear up your swabbing equipment after the patient has left and consider whether you have removed all trace of infection. You could consider asking the local infection control nurse (or infection control lead for the trust) to visit your clinic and give specific guidance to staff based on the facilities that you have. You should also ensure you (and other team members) are familiar with the local trust policies on infection control. An audit that assesses the team's knowledge and compliance with local policy guidelines would be valuable in assessing safety in practice.

# Collecting data to demonstrate your learning, competence, performance and standards of service delivery

## Example cycle of evidence 6.1

- Focus: clinical care
- Other relevant focus: relationships with patients

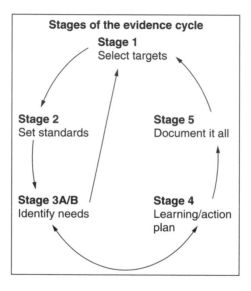

Stages of the evidence cycle

**Stage 1**
Select targets

**Stage 2**
Set standards

**Stage 5**
Document it all

**Stage 3A/B**
Identify needs

**Stage 4**
Learning/action plan

---

**Case study 6.2**

Miss Fret attends with 'lumps down below'. On examination, you find that she has several vulval warts and you refer her with a letter to the GUM clinic for screening (in case she has other STIs) and treatment. She contacts you again, even more distressed, as she cannot get an appointment at the GUM clinic for three weeks. You are annoyed that you will have to continue to organise her care.

---

This is just an example. Keep your task simple. You could choose three or four cycles of evidence to demonstrate your competence each year.

## Stage 1: Select your aspirations for good practice

The excellent nurse:

- provides or arranges investigations or treatment when necessary
- takes suitable and prompt action when required
- refers to another practitioner when indicated
- does not allow beliefs or values to influence the advice or treatment provided, or if beliefs are likely to affect patient management tells patients of their right to see another health professional who will be better able to serve their needs
- makes efficient use of resources, but records, reports and endeavours to rectify deficiencies in resources
- empowers patients to take decisions about their management.

## Stage 2: Set the standards for your outcomes

Outcomes might include:

- the way learning is applied
- a learnt skill
- a protocol
- a strategy that is implemented
- meeting recommended standards.

- Demonstrate consistent best practice in provision of investigation and treatment of suspected STIs in respect of availability and accessibility and clinical management.

## Stage 3A: Identify your learning needs

- Carry out a self-assessment of your knowledge about the investigation of STIs.
- Conduct a significant event audit e.g. a young woman who developed pelvic inflammatory disease three months after she failed to attend the GUM clinic after you gave her a referral letter.
- Keep a reflective diary capturing trends or comments relating to problems dealing with the sexual activity of young women.

## Stage 3B: Identify your service needs

Any of the needs assessment exercises in 3A may also reveal service needs.

- Record the pathway of care when young women with sexually related complaints consult you or other health professionals in the team.
- Collect data about access and arrangements for referral to the GUM clinic.

## Stage 4: Make and carry out a learning and action plan

- Compare your knowledge of the investigation and management of STIs in young women with an authoritative source you obtain and read.
- Prepare a draft practice guideline for the investigation and management of STIs.
- Obtain statistics about the workload and waiting times at the nearest GUM clinic and find out how you can make representations to try to improve the availability of services.
- Attend a workshop where you can compare your attitudes towards people with STIs with other people's to ensure that you are not behaving judgementally.

## Stage 5: Document your learning, competence, performance and standards of service delivery

- Collect feedback from the GUM clinic about service delivery.
- Collect feedback from other health professionals about your draft guidelines for the investigation and management of STIs.
- Extract information from your reflective diary about your greater understanding of young women's sexual behaviour and the changes you have made so that you feel that your attitude is not perceived as judgemental or defensive.

---

**Case study 6.2 continued**

Miss Fret is naturally anxious and unhappy about the management of her problems. You need to discuss with other team members how the situation can be best managed and then present Miss Fret with the options. The doctor advises that you take samples for investigation if Miss Fret is able to take them to the hospital laboratory to ensure their rapid transport. Once Miss Fret understands why this is important she is more than willing to do this. The results show that no other STI is present. You discuss the result with the doctor who advises regular painting of the warts with podophyllin which Miss Fret needs to wash off three hours after application. Miss Fret is happy to accept this option and successful treatment is therefore initiated promptly. You record in your portfolio the rewarding experience of working in partnership with the patient!

---

## Example cycle of evidence 6.2

- Focus: maintaining good medical practice
- Other relevant focus: working with colleagues

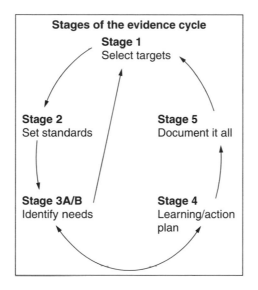

Stages of the evidence cycle
Stage 1 Select targets
Stage 2 Set standards
Stage 3A/B Identify needs
Stage 4 Learning/action plan
Stage 5 Document it all

---

**Case study 6.3**

Mrs Rabbit had been screened for STIs following a diagnosis of non-specific urethritis (NSU) in her current partner. You do not have access to urine testing in your area and EIA testing from a cervical swab did not pick up any infection. You explain to her that as a contact she should be treated, and decide to ask the doctor for a prescription for a seven day course of oxytetracyline. This is duly given. Later in the day, you notice Mrs Rabbit's name in the 'specimens' book and find that the healthcare assistant sent off a pregnancy test the previous day. You phone Mrs Rabbit and tell her not to take the tablets and to return to see you. You are annoyed with Mrs Rabbit for not telling you that she may be pregnant.

---

This is just an example. Keep your task simple. You could choose three or four cycles of evidence to demonstrate your competence each year.

## Stage 1: Select your aspirations for good practice

The excellent nurse:

- works with colleagues to monitor and maintain the quality of care provided
- is continually aware of patient safety
- takes part in regular and systematic clinical audits and makes improvements accordingly
- takes part in confidential enquiries, adverse event recognition and reporting, to help reduce risks to patients
- ensures systems are in place for adequate recording of ongoing investigations in patients' notes
- ensures that health professionals receive specimens for sending to pathology laboratories and that these are recorded in patients' notes at the time of sending.

## Stage 2: Set the standards for your outcomes

Outcomes might include:

- the way learning is applied
- a learnt skill
- a protocol
- a strategy that is implemented
- meeting recommended standards.

- Demonstrate consistent best practice for the management of test requests within the practice.
- Demonstrate consistent best practice in the prevention of harm to patients from potential prescribing errors.

## Stage 3A: Identify your learning needs

- Reflect on how best to change systems (receiving and sending specimens) so that the whole healthcare team is aware of the need for careful recording.
- Review your knowledge of the sensitivity and specificity of the tests (in this case in relation to sexual health) being used by your laboratory so that you understand fully the likelihood of a patient having a false positive or false negative result.
- Review the process for pregnancy testing – to ensure that patients are seen and counselled both before and after tests are sent.
- Reflect on the fact that you felt irritated with Mrs Rabbit when it was actually your responsibility to ask about possible pregnancy if this would affect treatment.

## Stage 3B: Identify your service needs

Any of the needs assessment exercises in 3A may also reveal service needs.

- Undertake a significant event audit where a prescribing error was made, with other clinicians in the team.
- Find out how requests for investigations are currently managed.
- Reflect on how you all inform other members of the team about what you have done, and how you find out what is happening. Do you need to increase your communication skills or use of internal email or make more effort to attend practice meetings?

## Stage 4: Make and carry out a learning and action plan

- Find out how other practices manage the results of investigations before making proposals at the practice meeting. Help to draw up standards that you propose which include that the date and time specimens are sent is recorded in the patient record.
- Raise the awareness of staff and patients to always ask about pregnancy. Make a poster to display for patients which advises on the importance of telling health professionals if they think they may be pregnant and reminding them to always ask whether a prescription is safe in pregnancy. Put a notice in a prominent place for clinicians to remind them: 'Have you considered whether this patient may be pregnant?'
- Revisit the guidelines on treatment of NSU and *Chlamydia* in women who are, or are not, pregnant.[7]
- Research the data about completion of treatment courses and decide whether an alternative treatment (such as azithromycin as a single dose) would be more cost-effective than oxytetracyline as a four times a day course for seven days.

## Stage 5: Document your learning, competence, performance and standards of service delivery

- Keep a copy of the standards of the record of how specimens will be received and sent off in the clinic.
- Record that you have laminated the posters you have made to ensure they do not deteriorate, and where you have put them on display.
- Keep a copy of your investigations into the management of *Chlamydia* in pregnancy.

- The successful completion of a specific education and training programme.
- All blood products should be assumed to be potentially injurious and handled accordingly. A protocol for needle-stick injuries is in place.[10,11]

### Stage 3A: Identify your learning needs

- Find or select a suitable questionnaire to use in an audit of health professionals' knowledge and attitudes about *Chlamydia* and HIV.
- Establish how to write the protocol for the research project and obtain ethical approval. Plan how you will analyse, collate and write up the findings.

### Stage 3B: Identify your service needs

Any of the needs assessment exercises in 3A may also reveal service needs.

- Establish the needs of both staff and patients for information, and of the staff for education and training.
- Manage the changeover from investigating *Chlamydia* to screening for it (*see* page 108).
- Determine how to manage the change to offering HIV testing to all as a routine and the confidentiality issues involved.

### Stage 4: Make and carry out a learning and action plan

- Refresh your research skills and bring them up to date.
- Understand the current requirements for ethical approval.
- Learn more about change management at a workshop.
- Work together with colleagues to examine the literature and draw up the protocol.
- Read a book or articles about completing research studies.
- Visit other clinics or surgeries already providing these services.

### Stage 5: Document your learning, competence, performance and standards of service delivery

- Record the progress with the project as the stages are worked through.
- Write up the project together with your colleagues when complete.
- Re-audit the level of knowledge amongst staff and patients.
- Keep a copy of research ethics approval and permission from the PCO to host the research.
- Keep a copy of the evaluation of the project.

---

**Case study 6.4 continued**

You soon abandon the idea of introducing screening for *Chlamydia* when you discover that you would have to wait for funding until the official Department of Health roll-out is funded in your area. You establish that there are low levels of knowledge amongst both patients and staff about HIV testing, and after an enthusiastic campaign of information and staff training you are able to introduce routine testing for HIV. The figures show a low level of uptake during the first six months, but a much better uptake by the second six months.

---

# References

1  Wakley G and Chambers R (2002) *Sexual Health Matters in Primary Care*. Radcliffe Medical Press, Oxford.

2  Department of Health (2001) *National Strategy for Sexual Health and HIV.* Department of Health, London.

3  The most recently available statistics on STIs are available from www.hpa.org.uk/infections/default.htm

4  Adler MW (1999) *ABC of Sexually Transmitted Diseases*. BMJ Publishing Group, London.

5  Godlee F (executive ed.) (2004) *Clinical Evidence Concise*. BMJ Publishing Group, London. www.clinicalevidence.com

6  Joint Formulary Committee (2004) *British National Formulary.* British Medical Association and Royal Pharmaceutical Society of Great Britain, London. Also at www.bnf.org

7  Godlee F (executive ed.) (2004) Chlamydia (uncomplicated, genital). In: *Clinical Evidence Concise.* **11**: 387–8.

8  Harvey J, Webb A and Mallinson H (2000) *Chlamydia trachomatis* screening in young people in Merseyside. *British Journal of Family Planning and Reproductive Health Care.* **26(4)**: 199–201.

9  Basarab A, Browning D, Lanham S and O'Connell S (2002) Pilot study to assess the presence of *Chlamydia trachomatis* in urine from 18–30-year-old males using EIA/IF and PCR. *British Journal of Family Planning and Reproductive Health Care.* **28(1)**: 36–7.

10 Board of Science and Education, British Medical Association (1998) *Bloodborne Viruses and Infection Control: a guide for health care professionals. Interactive CD ROM.* BMJ Books, London.

11 Department of Health (2000*) HIV Post-Exposure Prophylaxis: guidance from the UK Chief Medical Officers' Expert Advisory Group on AIDS*. Department of Health, London.

# Further reading and resources

• Avert (UK-based charity giving extensive AIDS information). www.avert.org

• CMO's expert advisory group report on *Chlamydia.* www.doh.gov.uk/assetRoot/04/06/22/64/04062264.pdf

- Department of Health National Strategy for Sexual Health and HIV. www.doh.gov.uk/assetRoot/04/05/89/45/04058945.pdf
- Genitourinary infections and GUM clinic list (British Association for Sexual Health and HIV). http://www.bashh.org
- Members of the BMA Foundation for AIDS (2002) *Take the HIV Test*. Medical Foundation for AIDS and Sexual Health, BMA House, Tavistock Square, London WC1H 9JP. www.medfash.org.uk
- Representatives of professional bodies and organisations producing guidelines. *Guidelines*: summarising clinical guidelines for primary care (latest issue). Medendium Group Publishing Ltd, Berkhamsted. And at www.eguidelines.co.uk. This gives you the source for the full guidelines for any particular condition.
- Scottish Intercollegiate Guidelines Network (SIGN). www.sign.ac.uk
- STI Online includes issues of *Sexually Transmitted Infections* published since 1967 and includes *Genitourinary Medicine* and *British Journal of Venereal Diseases*. http://sti.bmjjournals.com
- Wakley G, Cunnion M and Chambers R (2003) *Improving Sexual Health Advice*. Radcliffe Medical Press, Oxford.

# 7

# Managing infertility in primary care

Consultations for infertility can be complex and time consuming. This chapter explores investigations and treatment that can be undertaken within a primary or secondary care setting. It is recognised that, for most nurses working in primary care, the pathway of care that is outlined may be outside their usual scope of practice. However, a nurse who has sufficient interest in infertility can aspire to working at the level suggested in this chapter. Other nurses working in primary care may restrict their involvement with infertility to a very basic level. However, they will benefit from understanding the projected pathway of care on which patients may be embarking.

Patients are likely to have seen their GP before being referred to the nurse for support and investigations. Many nurses acquire considerable expertise in the management of infertility after initial involvement with patients to perform investigations (such as blood tests). Nurses are well known for their skills in listening and this is often a major requirement for patients who are unable to become pregnant easily. However, the ability to listen and empathise will not, by itself, help the patient to achieve a pregnancy so knowledge of the pathway through investigations and treatment is also required.

---

**Case study 7.1**

Mrs Brie is referred to see you by her GP. She is 32 years old and is very concerned that she has not achieved a pregnancy after trying for six months. The GP told Mrs Brie that this was not unusual but, in view of her distress, decides to send her to you for advice and preliminary investigations. You discover that Mrs Brie is a hairdresser who has a passion for soft cheeses and her husband is a sheep farmer, with a successfully expanding farm. Mrs Brie had a miscarriage three years earlier which she found very distressing and it has taken the couple some time to decide to try for a further pregnancy.

Mrs Brie has read on the Internet that dietary changes can have a major impact on fertility. You suspect Mrs Brie's passion for food may extend beyond soft cheese as she weighs 80 kg at a height of 1.6 m (BMI 31). Her menstrual cycle is regular at 28 days duration and she notices mid-cycle abdominal discomfort when her cervical mucus also seems more profuse.

---

# What issues you should cover

At the first consultation, it is important to outline the initial plan of care. This will help the couple to realise that they may not be in for a quick fix solution, but a methodical approach that will allow sufficient time to cover all aspects of treatment (including psychological support).

The first priority is to provide some prognostic information to reassure the couple that, although infertility is common, most couples will ultimately achieve a pregnancy. Secondly, it is important to take this opportunity for pre-pregnancy assessment to optimise the outlook for a healthy pregnancy and normal baby. Specific assessment regarding infertility should be commenced in a systematic fashion. An enthusiastic nurse with the ability to listen and interpret a patient's history can go a long way to establishing a diagnosis and steering a couple's management appropriately.[1] Arranging to see patients at monthly intervals for a 20-minute appointment should provide adequate time and satisfy them that care and treatment is ongoing.

Before arranging any tests, it is possible to give the couple useful prognostic information by considering their age, duration of infertility and any prior pregnancies.[2] Although it may be tempting to agree with the GP and reassure the couple that six months is too soon to worry, it is important first to establish how long the couple have been having intercourse without contraception. Couples may stop contraception without actively trying for a pregnancy and only regard the period of infertility as the time that they were actively trying for pregnancy. Although fertility declines with female age, at 32 years the outlook remains good. The influence of male age is much less marked. As the couple have achieved a pregnancy in the past, they are more likely to achieve a further pregnancy, even though the previous pregnancy did not lead to a baby.

The couple may find it useful for you to give them some idea of the average time to conception based on their circumstances. It is possible to calculate this from Table 7.1 or use the fertility calculator on the Repromed website.[3] Such calculators only provide a guide and individual circumstances may alter the prognosis. In this case, Mrs Brie is obese which may have an adverse influence even though she appears to be ovulating. She certainly should be encouraged to lose weight, setting realistic targets for weight loss.

Mrs Brie has particular risks from toxoplasmosis from the sheep and listeriosis from soft cheeses. It is important to explain this without causing undue alarm and suggest simple measures such as avoidance of soft cheeses, and the sheep, particularly at lambing time.

Modify the baseline cumulative pregnancy rate by applying each multiplication factor that applies to the couple, providing an individualised chance of pregnancy. For instance if a couple had one prior pregnancy, multiplying the baseline rate by 1.8 increases their cumulative live birth rate. If a couple had a prior pregnancy and had endometriosis, then multiply the baseline rate by 1.8 times 0.4.

**Table 7.1:** A guide to prognosis for pregnancy without fertility treatment[2]

| Average baseline prognosis | | Effects of prognostic factors | |
| --- | --- | --- | --- |
| Months | Cumulative live birth rate (%) | Prognostic factor | Multiplication factor |
| 3 | 4.2 | Prior pregnancy in partnership | 1.8 |
| 6 | 8.1 | Duration of infertility < 36 months | 1.7 |
| 12 | 14.3 | Female age < 30 years | 1.5 |
| 24 | 21.2 | Male defect | 0.5 |
| 36 | 25.2 | Endometriosis | 0.4 |
| | | Tubal defect | 0.5 |

# Initial infertility management

In February 2004, NICE released a comprehensive set of guidelines regarding the management of infertile couples including initial assessment and lifestyle advice.[4] Although the full guidelines may be a little daunting to work through, the summary document and management flow charts are a useful source of information for initial management. Pre-pregnancy tests include rubella immunity and routine cervical cytology. Pre-pregnancy advice covers stopping smoking, reducing alcohol intake, optimising weight and taking folic acid to reduce risk of neural tube defects. Ovulation is assessed by progesterone on day 21 of a 28 day cycle or later if the cycle is longer. Serum follicle stimulating hormone (FSH) and luteinising hormone (LH) at the start of the menstrual cycle can provide further useful information. A basic semen analysis is the first step in male investigations.

# Unexplained infertility

In many cases, initial assessment may uncover no specific cause for infertility. Even after comprehensive assessment, around one in four couples' infertility may be classified as 'unexplained'.[5]

---

**Case study 7.1 continued**

Mr and Mrs Brie return to see you with the results of the initial investigations that you have undertaken. Although initially following the miscarriage the couple had used condoms, they had stopped using any contraception over 14 months previously. Mrs Brie has joined a local dieting club, and since you last saw her six weeks previously she has lost 3 kg in weight. She has found this very difficult to achieve and wonders if she can have any treatment to help her to lose further weight.

---

It is important to provide the couple with reassurance and support explaining the likelihood of conception if they persevere. As the couple have over one year's infertility it is reasonable to suggest to the GP that they are referred to the local fertility clinic, particularly if the waiting list is long, as this secures their place in the 'queue' to be seen.

Weight reduction will not only benefit the chance of achieving a pregnancy but also will also improve the outlook for any pregnancy and have wider health benefits. The National electronic Library for Health provides guidance on weight reduction, including the place for medications,[6] and you could look at Chapter 4 again.

## Mixed tubal and male factor infertility

Multiple infertility factors commonly affect both the male and female. It is always important to manage a couple together and plan management that considers all factors. If you have access to hysterosalpingography this can provide very valuable information.

---

**Case study 7.2**

Mr and Mrs Fallow attend for explanation of the results of infertility tests that have been undertaken following 18 months of infertility at the ages of 37 and 39 years respectively. Although recent *Chlamydia* swabs had been negative, in the past Mrs Fallow had been treated for a bout of serious pelvic inflammatory disease. In view of the risk of tubal disease, the GP had arranged a hysterosalpingogram that revealed large bilateral hydrosalpinges. Mrs Fallow's *Chlamydia* serology is strongly positive but her other test results are unremarkable. Medical notes inform you that Mr Fallow's external genitalia appear normal on examination and semen analysis is: volume 2.5 ml, pH 7.4, concentration 14 million per ml, motility 40% normal, morphology 4% normal forms.

---

A hysterosalpingogram shows whether the uterus is normal and the tubes are patent. The investigation is usually undertaken in the X-ray department a few hours after taking pain relief, such as ibuprofen or paracetamol, to reduce discomfort. A radio-opaque dye is gradually introduced through the cervix and a series of X-ray pictures are taken as the uterus fills with dye, which gradually spills through the tubes if they are patent. Although a hysterosalpingogram may suggest a tube is blocked when it is not in around 10% of cases, they are reliable at identifying hydrosalpinges (fallopian tubes distended with fluid). For Mr and Mrs Fallow, the prognosis for successful tubal surgery is poor, partly because of the unfavourable factors of large hydrosalpinges and positive *Chlamydia* serology and because of the poor semen result (*see* Box 7.1 for normal values). Although the low borderline sperm count and reduced motility are of uncertain significance, the poor morphology (cell shape and structure) suggests a poor prognosis. If these results were confirmed with a repeat semen test, the optimal treatment would be assisted conception using intracytoplasmic sperm injection (ICSI). In ICSI, a single sperm is injected into the egg to enable fertilisation with very low sperm counts or with non-motile sperm.

It is known that large hydrosalpinges reduce pregnancy rates and increase miscarriage rates. Thus salpingectomy, or at least occlusion of the proximal fallopian tubes, should be considered before proceeding with ICSI. The couple need referral for specialist care and if they proceed with ICSI treatment, they will need to be tested for hepatitis B and C and HIV to comply with the Human Fertilisation and Embryology Authority's (HFEA's) guidelines on the storage of sperm and embryos.[7]

---

**Box 7.1:**    World Health Organization normal semen analysis values[8]

- Volume 2 ml or more
- pH 7.2 or more
- Sperm concentration >20 million per ml
- Total sperm number 40 or more million sperm per ejaculate
- Motility >50%
- Morphology 15% or more normal forms
- Sperm antibody tests:
  - immunobead test <50% motile sperms bound to beads
  - mixed antiglobulin reaction (MAR) test <50% motile sperms bound

---

# Male factor infertility

Around one in four infertile couples has evidence of male factor problems, and around one in 20 shows a complete absence of any sperm. Nurses working with infertility need to consider how to manage the couple following the semen result, particularly as the couple may become very distressed and even angry if the news is bad. It is useful to provide couples with basic statistics about infertility and an explanation about varying causes, which they can take away and read before the next appointment. This should impress on them that infertility can be a male or female problem (or a combination!) so that they are prepared for problems relating to either of them.

---

**Case study 7.3**

Mr and Mrs Baron have completed basic infertility investigations and have arranged an appointment with you to review their results. Mrs Baron is a healthy 31 year old with no known medical problems, although she has a cousin who has cystic fibrosis. Mr Baron takes a beta-blocker for hypertension, which is well controlled and he is otherwise well. The results of the investigations are given overleaf.

---

**Mrs Baron**
- Rubella antibodies detected confirming immunity
- LH 3.1 IU/l FSH 4 IU/l
- Progesterone 38 nmol/l
- *Chlamydia* serology negative

**Mr Baron: semen analysis**
- Volume 3.2 ml
- pH 7.2
- Liquefaction: normal
- No sperm were observed

At the initial consultation, the GP had not examined Mr Baron, but in view of the above discovery you would now expect the GP to examine him. He has a moderate sized varicocele on the left-hand side and his vas deferens on either side cannot be positively identified.

At the initial infertility consultation, you will not have adequate time for a complete assessment, thus it is reasonable to defer the male genitalia examination until the result of the semen analysis is known. The main priority is to identify lumps that could be testicular cancer and necessitate urgent referral. Checking testicular volume and the presence of the vas deferens can provide very helpful information. If you are unfamiliar with this examination then it may be worth arranging to sit in on a clinic with a local specialist to learn more. There are conflicting views on the importance of varicoceles in male infertility, but the treatment of varicoceles is unlikely to be beneficial if the sperm count is very low.

Drugs may affect sperm production and/or ability to achieve intravaginal ejaculation. It is possible for beta-blockers to cause impotence but they are not associated with azoospermia. If you encounter a problem in a man on medication, check for possible side-effects in the *British National Formulary*.[9]

Azoospermia may be caused by chromosome abnormalities hence it is advisable to check his karyotype and screen for Y deletions with a blood test. The azoospermia could be caused by congenital bilateral absence of the vas deferens, which is associated with the carriage of cystic fibrosis mutations. In view of this genetic risk to the child, it is important to counsel the couple about whether they wish to have screening for carriage of cystic fibrosis mutations.

The treatment options open to the couple are donor insemination i.e. insemination using semen donated by an anonymous male, or surgical sperm retrieval followed by ICSI. Surgical sperm retrieval refers to a range of surgical procedures to collect sperm directly from the epidydimis or testes. Both surgical sperm retrieval followed by ICSI and donor insemination are effective, with pregnancy rates of 30% for one cycle of ICSI or about three cycles of donor insemination. If there is an obstructive cause for azoospermia, it is usually possible to collect sperm surgically, but if there is a primary testicular problem then no sperm may be obtained. A low testicular volume and blood tests such as high FSH help predict the risk of not collecting sperm – the smaller the testis and the higher the FSH, the less likely that it will be possible to collect sperm.

# Ovulatory infertility

Irregular menstruation is a useful pointer to ovulatory dysfunction, which may be very responsive to appropriate treatment. However, further tests are required to clarify the cause of irregular periods.

---

**Case study 7.4**

Mr and Mrs Nimble are a young couple who have completed basic infertility investigations. Mrs Nimble is a slim aerobics instructor who has erratic periods occurring at anything from 4- to 10-week intervals. In view of this, the GP has arranged a few additional tests and the results are given below.

- LH 14 IU/l
- FSH 4 IU/l
- Thyroid stimulating hormone (TSH) 2 nmol/l
- Prolactin 240 mU/l
- Sex hormone binding globulin (SHBG) 20 nmol/l
- Testosterone 3.2 nmol/l

---

The most common cause for irregular menstruation is polycystic ovarian syndrome (PCOS). Mrs Nimble has the typical biochemical features of a raised LH, raised LH/ FSH ratio (above 2.5), raised testosterone and lower SHBG levels. However, in many patients, this is not the case and expert opinion is divided on the precise definition of PCOS, including the role and appearance of ultrasonography of the ovaries. Although hyperprolactinaemia is an infrequent cause of irregular menstruation, it is important to check prolactin levels, as one of the causes is pituitary microadenoma and specialist referral would then be appropriate.

The first step in the management of anovulatory PCOS is weight reduction if the woman is obese, but, as with this patient, not everyone with PCOS is obese. Opinion is divided regarding initial medication. First-line treatment used to be anti-oestrogen therapy with clomiphene, but concerns about the risk of multiple pregnancies and ovarian cancer now make this approach less attractive and other treatments are of unknown effectiveness.[10] Insulin-sensitising agents such as metformin are increasingly used.[11]

# Collecting data to demonstrate your learning, competence, performance and standards of service delivery

## Example cycle of evidence 7.1

- Focus: clinical care

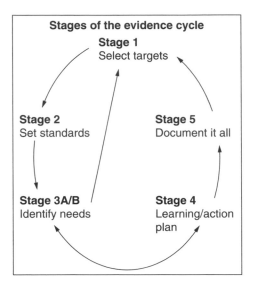

**Stages of the evidence cycle**

**Stage 1**
Select targets

**Stage 2**
Set standards

**Stage 5**
Document it all

**Stage 3A/B**
Identify needs

**Stage 4**
Learning/action plan

---

**Case study 7.5**

Mrs Lack pops in to see you in the treatment room while you are preparing for a clinic and asks you about her preliminary infertility investigations. She has read an article on the Internet suggesting that she could improve her fertility by altering her diet. She asks if the result of her husband's semen test is available yet. You look up the results in your consulting room and discover the semen test revealed a complete absence of sperm. You tell Mrs Lack that you need to speak to the GP. You discuss with the GP the confidentiality issues around giving Mr Lack's semen result to his wife. You both agree that the results should be conveyed personally to Mr Lack with due sensitivity.

Checking the medical record, you note the management plan is for the *couple* to return for a follow-up consultation to discuss the results when they are all available. Accordingly, you ask Mrs Lack to make a joint appointment explaining that discussion of results will occur then.

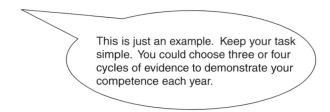

This is just an example. Keep your task simple. You could choose three or four cycles of evidence to demonstrate your competence each year.

## Stage 1: Select your aspirations for good practice

The excellent nurse:
- keeps comprehensive records outlining the management plan and information given to patients, including details of how results will be followed up and patients informed of results
- ensures that information is conveyed sensitively and appropriately, respecting confidentiality.

## Stage 2: Set the standards for your outcomes

> Outcomes might include:
>
> - the way learning is applied
> - a learnt skill
> - a protocol
> - a strategy that is implemented
> - meeting recommended standards.

- Demonstrate consistent best practice in providing assessment and treatment for infertile couples.
- Demonstrate consistent best practice in keeping good patient medical records in that a management plan was recorded at the end of each consultation for infertility.

## Stage 3A: Identify your learning needs

- Consider if you know how to interpret the semen results that come from your local service, and what information needs to be given to patients with the various types of result.
- When recording data such as a semen analysis, undertake an audit that highlights whether notes included a check to show that the patient has an appointment to discuss the result.
- Reflect on whether you know the current views on the link between diet and infertility.

## Stage 3B: Identify your service needs

Any of the needs assessment exercises in 3A may also reveal service needs.

- Track what happens to basic semen reports when they are received by the practice.
- Check whether the local laboratory follows WHO guidelines and the results they produce are consistent with WHO normal values.[8]
- Discuss with nursing and medical colleagues the best way to give patients the results of sensitive tests such as semen analysis.
- Compare the management of patients in your practice with the NICE guidelines.[4]
- Audit 10 records of patients consulting for infertility to determine if a management plan is recorded at each attendance.

## Stage 4: Make and carry out a learning and action plan

- Read about semen tests, causes of abnormality and subsequent management options.
- Write a simple handout for patients, going through the significance of the results of the infertility tests you arrange and discuss this with colleagues.
- Meet with other staff to talk through aspects of confidentiality of medical records. Consider producing (or updating) confidentiality guidelines including reference to relevant resources.[12,13]
- Prepare summary guidance for management of infertility based on the NICE guidelines and other local recommendations, for a resource available to all clinical staff on the computer desktop.

## Stage 5: Document your learning, competence, performance and standards of service delivery

- Track your infertility consultations over a year and keep a copy of your review of how they were assessed and patients informed of results.
- Record the feedback from other health professionals about your approach to infertility management.
- File your patient infertility results information sheet in your portfolio.
- Keep a copy of the summary guidance for the management of infertility that is available to all clinical staff.

> **Case study 7.5 continued**
>
> Mr and Mrs Lack return to the GP surgery the following week, when you have had time to discuss the management of azoospermia and obtain all the test results. The couple was relieved that you gave them this news together and had a clear plan of action, starting with a repeat semen test for confirmation of the results. Having heard this news, they were less interested in the role of diet in infertility but were pleased that you were aware of the subject, providing them with simple advice and reassurance.

# Example cycle of evidence 7.2

• Focus: maintaining good medical practice

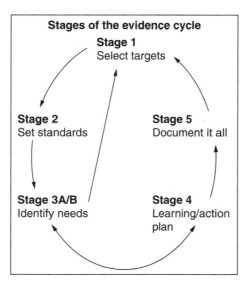

> **Case study 7.6**
>
> Mrs Jumble has been referred to you for support relating to her infertility. She has a history of irregular menstruation and this has persisted despite taking clomiphene for the past six months. The GP feels that Mrs Jumble has become overly dependent on him. She is visiting the surgery almost every week asking for pregnancy tests and consultations apparently result in Mrs Jumble weeping. The GP finds this difficult to cope with and feels he doesn't have the time to listen to Mrs Jumble's repeated anxieties relating to her infertility.

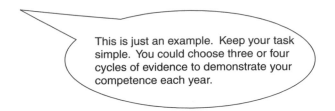

This is just an example. Keep your task simple. You could choose three or four cycles of evidence to demonstrate your competence each year.

### Stage 1: Select your aspirations for good practice

The excellent nurse will:

- be aware of the investigations that should have been undertaken in line with best practice
- determine Mrs Jumble's understanding of her situation
- act as the patient's advocate.

### Stage 2: Set the standards for your outcomes

Outcomes might include:

- the way learning is applied
- a learnt skill
- a protocol
- a strategy that is implemented
- meeting recommended standards.

- Ensure that Mrs Jumble has the correct investigations in line with best practice.
- Demonstrate best practice in patient education by supplying information appropriate to Mrs Jumble's situation.

### Stage 3A: Identify your learning needs

- Contact the services you have identified as potentially helpful and find out what they have to offer. Make notes relating to the type of help and support that can be offered, including details of local contacts.
- Find out what investigations Mrs Jumble has had and check that these are in line with best practice. Discuss any apparent omissions in care with the GP in order that appropriate tests may be initiated.

### Stage 3B: Identify your service needs

Any of the needs assessment exercises in 3A may also reveal service needs.

- Discover in what ways other staff provide psychological support for patients.
- Discuss with colleagues and patients whether it would be helpful to put patients in the same situation in touch with one another to form self-help groups. Approach the individuals and gain their permission to give out contact details if they feel able to help others.

## Stage 4: Make and carry out a learning and action plan

- Perform a literature search on psychological support for patients with infertility to determine effective care. Share this information with the GP who evidently felt ill-equipped to deal with this situation.
- Obtain a list of helpful resources and circulate these to colleagues, explaining that you have checked out and commented on what is on offer.
- Put together a variety of information packs that you are able to loan or give to patients.

## Stage 5: Document your learning, competence, performance and standards of service delivery

- Incorporate the new information in the guidelines for the use in your practice by all the clinicians.
- Re-audit the management of PCOS to confirm that the modern management guidelines are being followed.
- Keep a list of the resources and information sources that you have identified.
- Record your reflections on the value of the support that you can offer Mrs Jumble and patients like her.

---

**Case study 7.6 continued**

Mrs Jumble presents three months later. She tells you that she meets up with a local support group twice a month when she has an opportunity to offload her feelings about not being pregnant yet. As a result, she feels that she does not have to burden all her friends and relatives quite as much. This has made her a little more relaxed at home. She remains optimistic about becoming pregnant and she tells you what she will ask the consultant to do next if her current treatment of clomiphene does not work. She says that she feels she is becoming 'quite an expert' and you are pleased to see how empowered she now appears.

---

# Example cycle of evidence 7.3

• Focus: relationships with patients

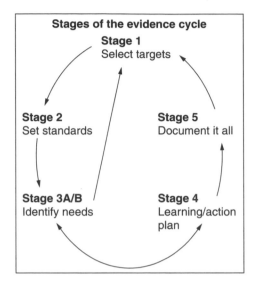

**Stages of the evidence cycle**

**Stage 1**
Select targets

**Stage 2**
Set standards

**Stage 5**
Document it all

**Stage 3A/B**
Identify needs

**Stage 4**
Learning/action
plan

---

**Case study 7.7**

Mr and Mrs Lament attend to discuss their infertility tests. Mrs Lament's hysterosalpingogram has revealed large bilateral hydrosalpinges and her husband has a low sperm count. You start to explain that they have serious barriers to a pregnancy and they may require assisted conception treatment. Mr Lament enquires whether there is anything he can do to improve his fertility. Mrs Lament wonders why she has developed tubal problems when she was never aware of any pelvic infection in the past. As the consultation progresses and you start to explain that it may be advisable to remove the fallopian tubes before considering assisted conception treatment, Mrs Lament starts to cry.

---

This is just an example. Keep your task simple. You could choose three or four cycles of evidence to demonstrate your competence each year.

## Stage 1: Select your aspirations for good practice

The excellent nurse:

- provides patients with sufficient information to make choices about their management
- provides support for patients faced with difficult decisions and frustrations.

## Stage 2: Set the standards for your outcomes

Outcomes might include:

- the way learning is applied
- a learnt skill
- a protocol
- a strategy that is implemented
- meeting recommended standards.

- Demonstrate best practice in providing information to patients.
- Development of your counselling skills through appropriate courses or through mentorship with a suitable peer or senior colleague.

## Stage 3A: Identify your learning needs

- Self-assess your learning needs about breaking bad news – after an occasion when you had to do that.
- Complete a quiz in a nursing or medical newspaper about interpretation and results of infertility tests.

## Stage 3B: Identify your service needs

Any of the needs assessment exercises in 3A may also reveal service needs.

- Get feedback from colleagues and staff for whom you are responsible, as to whether you recognise and are sensitive to patients' feelings and have strategies to deal with distressed patients.
- Participate in a 360° feedback exercise arranged by the practice team – focusing on breaking bad news and enabling patients to make informed decisions about treatment.

*Stage 4: Make and carry out a learning and action plan*

- Ask a colleague who has done a breaking bad news course to facilitate role-play scenarios of difficult patient–staff interactions, where the patient is very distressed, at an in-house educational session for the team.
- Attend a course on breaking bad news.[14]
- Sit in a clinic on one or more occasions with an infertility specialist and ask lots of questions about infertility tests and treatment.

*Stage 5: Document your learning, competence, performance and standards of service delivery*

- Keep records of your interactions with other distressed patients (suitably anonymised) and record your conclusions about your improvement in your reflective diary.
- Keep your notes from your attendance at the course.
- Keep copies of the feedback from others in the team.

---

**Case study 7.7 continued**

You feel that you have identified the need for time in dealing with infertile couples when breaking bad news, and will consider how best to handle this in your surgery.

---

# Example cycle of evidence 7.4

- Focus: working with colleagues
- Other relevant focus: teaching and training

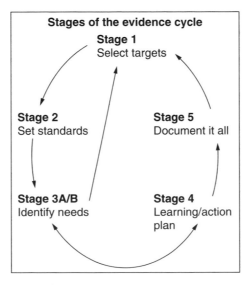

**Stages of the evidence cycle**

**Stage 1**
Select targets

**Stage 2**
Set standards

**Stage 5**
Document it all

**Stage 3A/B**
Identify needs

**Stage 4**
Learning/action plan

---

**Case study 7.8**

Eva Lait is 26 years old and comes to the cytology clinic to have a routine cervical smear taken. When you ask her about contraception Eva states that she has been trying to get pregnant for the past six months, and is dismayed that this hasn't happened yet. She then mentions that she has had a milky discharge from her breasts and has had no periods for four months. Eva tells you that she spoke to the doctor about this on the phone. He told her that as she was attending for a cervical smear the nurse would advise about this problem.

---

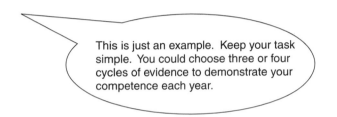

This is just an example. Keep your task simple. You could choose three or four cycles of evidence to demonstrate your competence each year.

## *Stage 1: Select your aspirations for good practice*

The excellent nurse:

- helps to educate patients
- uses robust evidence to manage care effectively.

## *Stage 2: Set the standards for your outcomes*

---

Outcomes might include:

- the way learning is applied
- a learnt skill
- a protocol
- a strategy that is implemented
- meeting recommended standards.

---

- Demonstrate skills in diagnosis and treatment planning.

## *Stage 3A: Identify your learning needs*

- Check that your knowledge relating to amenorrhoea and galactorrhoea is up to date by accessing best practice guidelines.

- Think about the explanation you would give to a patient who asked why this was happening. Rehearse this explanation with a senior colleague (this may be a doctor or senior nurse) to check that it is accurate and clear.
- Note down the investigations that should be undertaken for these presenting signs and symptoms and ensure that you know what normal results should be, and what abnormal results signify.
- Discuss with the doctor what action and advice he expected you to give and reflect on whether this is reasonable.

## Stage 3B: Identify your service needs

> Any of the needs assessment exercises in 3A may also reveal service needs.

- Check with the practice team what expectations they have of the advice and actions you can reasonably be expected to give about galactorrhoea and infertility.

## Stage 4: Make and carry out a learning and action plan

- Visit the local nursing library to find out more about these conditions. Read the relevant data in several texts or articles written within the last few years.
- Arrange a meeting or clinical supervision session with other nurses to talk about your new-found knowledge and share experiences relating to treatment of patients with these symptoms.
- Devise a teaching package that can be used for either nurses or patients to explain the physiological processes leading to galactorrhoea and amenorrhoea.
- Suggest a journal club to your colleagues and offer to launch the first session with your review of an article relating to this subject.

## Stage 5: Document your learning, competence, performance and standards of service delivery

- Keep a copy in your portfolio of the teaching package you have devised.
- Make notes relating to the discussion that took place at your journal club meeting. Distribute these to those who attended and any other interested colleagues and keep a copy in your portfolio.
- Write a short reflective piece identifying what you have learnt from this encounter.

---

**Case study 7.8 continued**

At the end of the consultation, the patient feels happy that her condition has been explained so thoroughly. You feel that your knowledge has increased and your ability to explain about galactorrhoea is enhanced.

---

# References

1  Jenkins JM, Corrigan L and Chambers R (2002) *Infertility Matters in Healthcare.* Radcliffe Medical Press, Oxford.

2  Collins JA, Burrows EA and Willan AR (1995) The prognosis for live birth among untreated infertile couples. *Fertility and Sterility.* **64**: 22–8.

3  www.repromed.org.uk/book/content/Fertility_Calculator.htm

4  www.nice.org.uk/cat.asp?c=104435

5  Cahill DJ and Wardle PG (2002) Management of infertility. *British Medical Journal.* **325**: 28–32. http://bmj.com/cgi/content/full/325/7354/28?maxtoshow

6  www.nelh.nhs.uk

7  Human Fertilisation and Embryology Authority (2001) *Screening of Patients. Letter 6th June 2001 from HFEA chairman to all IVF clinics.* Human Fertilisation and Embryology Authority, London.

8  World Health Organization (1999) WHO *Laboratory Manual for the Examination of Human Semen and Sperm–Cervical Mucus Interaction* (4e). Cambridge University Press, Cambridge.

9  www.bnf.org

10  www.clinicalevidence.com

11  www.rcog.org.uk/mainpages.asp?PageID=1413

12  www.informationcommissioner.gov.uk

13  http://www.nmc-uk.org

14  Kate Grimes, Programme Leader: Transforming Healthcare Delivery, King's Healthcare NHS Trust. (2000) Breaking bad news. *Bandolier.* **8**: 6. www.jr2.ox.ac.uk/bandolier/ImpAct/imp08/i8-6.html

# 8

# Vaginal bleeding problems in primary care

Nurses in primary care, with an interest in women's health, encounter women with a wide range of vaginal bleeding problems. This chapter focuses on some of the more common problems that may be encountered relating to menstruation and provides references to more in-depth information available.

---

**Case study 8.1**

Mrs Flud is a 43-year-old woman who is distraught because her periods have become increasingly heavy and troublesome over the last five months. Her menstrual cycle remains regular and she had a normal cervical smear six months earlier. She feels tired all the time and fed up with her heavy periods. However, she does not want a hysterectomy and she is concerned that if she seeks medical help she will be forced to lose her uterus.

---

# What issues you should cover

## Menorrhagia

Before considering treatment, it is important to consider whether there may be any significant underlying pathology. The clinical management of menorrhagia is summarised in Figure 8.1.[1]

A study of a cohort of women in Oxford up to the end of 1989 suggested that around one in five women in the UK had a hysterectomy before 55 years of age.[2] In many of these cases the uterus was normal, particularly in women who had previous pregnancies. However, improvements in conservative management of menorrhagia mean that there are now many options to improve Mrs Flud's heavy periods without a hysterectomy.[3] Figure 8.2 provides guidelines for management using a variety of options. As part of the nurse's role is to act as the patient's advocate, it is important to be aware of all the treatment options in order to discuss these with patients. The levonorgestrel intrauterine system (IUS) is a good method that has been shown to produce up to a 90% reduction in menstrual loss.[4] The IUS also reduces dysmenorrhoea and provides contraception[5] (*see* Chapter 5 for further details).

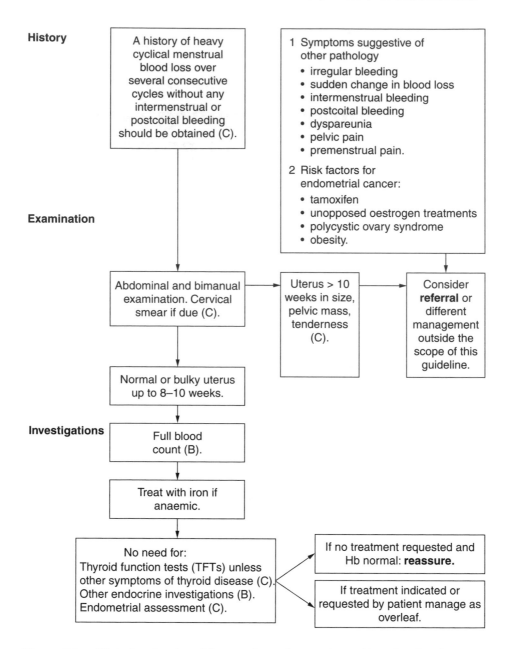

**History**

A history of heavy cyclical menstrual blood loss over several consecutive cycles without any intermenstrual or postcoital bleeding should be obtained (C).

1  Symptoms suggestive of other pathology
   - irregular bleeding
   - sudden change in blood loss
   - intermenstrual bleeding
   - postcoital bleeding
   - dyspareunia
   - pelvic pain
   - premenstrual pain.

2  Risk factors for endometrial cancer:
   - tamoxifen
   - unopposed oestrogen treatments
   - polycystic ovary syndrome
   - obesity.

**Examination**

Abdominal and bimanual examination. Cervical smear if due (C).

Uterus > 10 weeks in size, pelvic mass, tenderness (C).

Consider **referral** or different management outside the scope of this guideline.

Normal or bulky uterus up to 8–10 weeks.

**Investigations**

Full blood count (B).

Treat with iron if anaemic.

No need for:
Thyroid function tests (TFTs) unless other symptoms of thyroid disease (C).
Other endocrine investigations (B).
Endometrial assessment (C).

If no treatment requested and Hb normal: **reassure.**

If treatment indicated or requested by patient manage as overleaf.

**Figure 8.1:**  Clinical evaluation of the complaint of menorrhagia (reproduced with permission from the Royal College of Obstetricians and Gynaecologists).[1] Level of evidence: (A), based on randomised controlled trials; (B), based on other robust experimental or observational studies; (C), based on more limited evidence but the advice relies on expert opinion and has the endorsement of respected authorities.

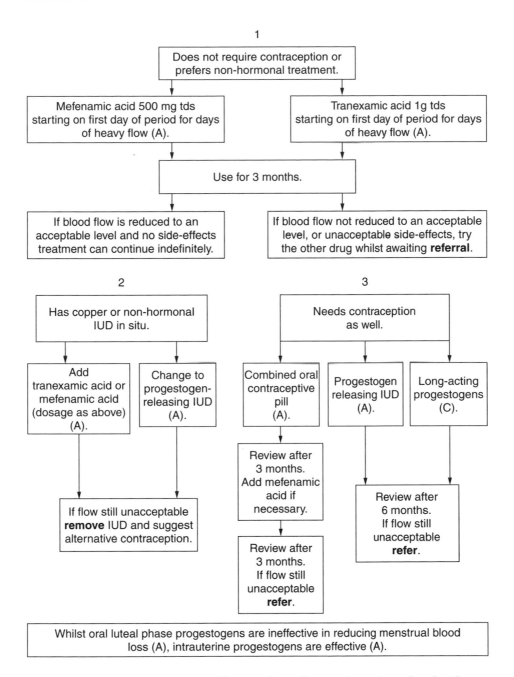

**Figure 8.2:** Medical management of the complaint of menorrhagia (reproduced with permission from the Royal College of Obstetricians and Gynaecologists).[1] This figure outlines different approaches to treatment depending on whether the patient does not require contraception (1), is using non-hormonal contraception (2) or requires contraception (3). Evidence levels (A), (B) and (C) are the same as in Figure 8.1.

Even if medical therapy is unsuccessful, there are several new techniques to reduce or remove the endometrium (ablation) without taking out the uterus, producing satisfactory results in 80–90% of patients.[6] Sometimes nurses working in primary care can feel far removed from the fast-moving innovations that seem to be occurring in secondary care. Arranging a visit to your local gynaecological outpatients department can be enormously helpful in updating you on new methods. Many gynaecological departments will have a clinical nurse specialist whom you could contact. Visiting a department to learn about techniques used and seeing the equipment used will enable you to provide the women you see in primary care with a better understanding of what they may encounter if they are referred to the hospital. Check on the local availability and gynaecologists' experience with new techniques such as balloon systems delivering local hot water to the endometrium, devices delivering radiofrequency, thermal energy or electromagnetic energy in the uterine cavity and endometrial cryoablation. Even if Mrs Flud has symptomatic fibroids, uterine artery embolisation conserving the uterus has been shown to provide a satisfactory result in around 90% of cases.[7]

---

**Case study 8.1 continued**

Mrs Flud has no indicators of serious pathology but a full blood count shows a haemoglobin level of 10.2 g/dl indicating that she is mildly iron deficient, and she starts taking some oral iron. After discussion of the options, she decides to have a levonorgestrel IUS fitted. She needs support to continue with it, as her menstrual loss is not immediately improved. You encourage her to keep a diary recording her bleeding pattern, with a note of how heavy the bleeding is, to demonstrate whether this is improving. After six months of use she is pleased to find that her periods are much more manageable.

---

# Dysmenorrhoea and endometriosis

Miss Payne's history suggests endometriosis, although it is not possible to make a definitive diagnosis of endometriosis without visualising it, usually by laparoscopy for

---

**Case study 8.2**

Following a particularly painful period, 22-year-old Miss Payne visits you complaining that she is unable to cope with her periods any longer. Over the last few months, she has found that simple analgesia has become progressively less effective, although she is relieved that between her periods she has no significant discomfort. She is not in a relationship at present, but she wishes to have children in the future, and she is concerned because her elder sister has recently had a total abdominal hysterectomy and her tubes and ovaries removed for endometriosis.

pelvic deposits or ultrasound examination for endometriomas. Alternative explanations for her symptoms of excessive pain should be considered. These might include idiopathic dysmenorrhoea, irritable bowel syndrome and pelvic inflammatory disease. Ask her about her bowels and symptoms of infection. Vaginal examination should be undertaken, recognising that this may uncover significant tenderness if there are deposits of endometriosis present or an enlarged ovary if it contains an endometrioma. If a woman is not trying to conceive and vaginal examination reveals no abnormality, symptomatic relief may be attempted. Discuss with her whether she would be happy to use the combined oral contraceptive pill (monthly or tricycling by taking three packets sequentially without a break). Taking combined oral contraceptives with non-steroidal anti-inflammatory drugs during her periods may help significantly.

However, if the pain is not controlled by this treatment, or if the patient is anxious, then it would be appropriate for her to be referred to a gynaecologist for a laparoscopy to establish the diagnosis. Endometriosis may be controlled by progestogens, danazol or gonadotrophin releasing hormone (GnRH) agonists. If GnRH agonists are used for any length of time, add-back oestrogen therapy is required to prevent postmenopausal problems such as low bone density.[8] Surgical treatment by ablation or excision laparoscopically or at laparotomy may prove necessary for control of the pain.[9] Further information on the investigation and management of endometriosis can be found on the Royal College of Obstetricians and Gynaecologists' website.[10]

---

**Case study 8.2 continued**

Miss Payne returns after taking three packs of a combined oral contraceptive and is obviously unhappy. Despite an improvement in the pain, she is still very anxious that her future fertility will be affected. You discuss her case with the GP who agrees to refer her on to a specialist.

---

# Threatened miscarriage of pregnancy

Nurses working in primary care often receive enquiries relating to early pregnancy. However, for most nurses, management of pregnancy-related concerns would fall outside their scope of practice. Patients with bleeding at any stage of pregnancy should be referred urgently to the GP or midwife. However, women who have had recurrent miscarriage frequently use nurses as a source of support. Recurrent

---

**Case study 8.3**

Following an anxious night, Mrs Loss phones you for advice. She has had light vaginal bleeding but no pain at eight weeks' gestation in her second pregnancy. In her first pregnancy, she had miscarried at seven weeks and she is very concerned that she may miscarry again.

miscarriage is defined as the loss of at least three pregnancies and affects one in 100 women. Couples may be distraught even after two miscarriages, particularly if associated with infertility and increased female age. Staying up to date with current treatments enables you to explain various treatment pathways to patients and help them to feel that they have had the appropriate care and investigations. Invite local community midwives to team meetings twice a year or so in order to discuss any new advances in treatments for early pregnancy loss. They may also benefit from hearing about your involvement with patients who have miscarried, and hearing the issues that patients raise while grieving for their loss.

---

**Case study 8.3 continued**

Mrs Loss comes to see you several weeks later and tells you that she miscarried again. She is angry with the GP who said that nothing could be done to save the pregnancy, as she has since read on the Internet that progesterone is effective in preventing miscarriages. She feels that if she had been given progesterone she would still be pregnant.

---

It is common for patients to try and manipulate nurses to side with them against doctors. However tempting on occasions, this can only produce a lack of professionalism that is unhelpful to all concerned. Although health professionals should encourage patients to research treatments for their condition, they should also be aware that information obtained by patients may not have been properly critiqued. It is often out of date, or biased by personal experience. The low progesterone level found in pregnancies that go on to become miscarriages is a sign that the pregnancy is already failing. Many studies have been done to investigate whether giving progesterone can prevent this loss, but the end result has been no difference between women who are given progesterone and those who are not. There was a review of evidence and consensus statement from the British Royal College of Obstetricians and Gynaecologists. The current guidelines relating to early pregnancy loss state that the value of progesterone to reduce the risk of miscarriage remains unproven and is likely to fall into the category of procedures which are particularly wasteful of resources and appear to be of little or no benefit.[11] At present, progesterone should only be used in this condition in the context of research studies.

Nurses dealing with patients who have suffered miscarriage should also be aware that a grieving reaction occurs that follows the typical bereavement response. This will include anger, and it is often directed at doctors or the hospital. Nurses can support patients to enable them to move through the cycle of grief to reach acceptance. Say you are sorry about what has happened and about their pain. Avoid saying that you know how they feel – everyone feels differently – or saying anything that implies judgement about their feelings. It is important not to tell them what they should feel or do. Never say, or imply, that they can always have another baby, or try to find something positive about the loss such as a moral lesson, closer family ties, or ability to finish a course of study or work. There will be many feelings of doubt and guilt already, so help the person to accept that miscarriage is common and about one in 36 women will have two miscarriages due to nothing more than chance.

It is also important to recognise when the grief process becomes stuck at a particular stage. This may require referral onto a community psychiatric nurse for assessment or onto a voluntary organisation that is able to offer specialised and intensive support. It is useful to keep an up-to-date list of telephone numbers for local agencies that provide support for patients following miscarriage or termination of pregnancy. Contact details can often be obtained from national organisations.[12]

## Suspected ectopic pregnancy

The diagnosis is unclear at this stage. Although Mrs Burst has presented for an IUD check, a vaginal examination is entirely inappropriate. It could prove to be extremely risky if she has an ectopic pregnancy on the threshold of rupture. It is therefore essential to undertake a pregnancy test, using a sensitive pregnancy test urine dipstick. If the pregnancy test is positive, then urgent referral to the first available doctor is required in order to arrange gynaecological admission. If the test is negative, you will need to think further. A differential diagnosis of complications from ovarian cysts or acute pelvic inflammatory disease should be considered.

---

**Case study 8.4**

Mrs Burst comes to see you asking for an IUD check. She tells you that she has had lower abdominal pain for the last few days, which is severe on occasions, and remembers you telling her that this should always be investigated promptly in case it indicates early signs of infection. Her coil was inserted 18 months ago, and although she complains that her periods are still irregular and usually heavy, she is happy with it. Her last period started two days earlier, but had been 12 days late and was unusually light. However, as her periods have always tended to be irregular Mrs Burst had thought nothing of this. You note that she has a mild pyrexia and abdominal examination reveals lower abdominal tenderness.

---

It is often very difficult to diagnose ectopic pregnancy in the early stages. A period may not have been missed and lower intermittent abdominal pain could be almost anything. It is frequently put down to irritable bowel syndrome, gastroenteritis or a urinary infection. Think about the possibility of an ectopic pregnancy, especially if there has been any change in the nature of the last episode of bleeding. The bleeding is often described as being like prune juice. Carry out a sensitive pregnancy test, and perhaps arrange for an early pregnancy scan. These actions help to improve the chances of an early diagnosis before an ectopic pregnancy leaks causing shoulder-tip pain as well as abdominal pain, or ruptures causing sudden collapse. If early diagnosis can be achieved before rupture of the tube and the appropriate facilities provided, less invasive treatment can be offered. Keyhole surgery or treatment with drugs can facilitate a speedier recovery and may increase the woman's chance of future fertility. The pregnancy is always going to be lost if it is ectopic but it may be possible for the surgeon, using laparoscopy, to cut the tube and remove the pregnancy, leaving the tube intact. Alternatively, in some centres a new treatment is offered using methotrexate to destroy the pregnancy. The drug can either be injected directly under ultrasound or laparoscopic guidance of a needle into the ectopic pregnancy or injected into a muscle, and then absorbed into the bloodstream to reach the ectopic pregnancy, avoiding any damage to the fallopian tube.

---

**Case study 8.4 continued**

After reviewing Mrs Burst with the doctor, admission is arranged. You stay with her until the ambulance arrives, in case her condition deteriorates acutely if an ectopic pregnancy were to rupture. You discuss with her what investigations she might have (e.g. ultrasound, laparoscopy) to prepare her. You check her blood pressure and pulse and ensure that the patient is handed over to the ambulance staff before you leave her.

---

## Amenorrhoea

If this information is not volunteered you may need to ask specifically about the following points.

- Establish with Miss Little that her mother does mean that she has *never* had a period, not just none for two months! It is possible, too, for ovulation to occur before a first period. Always think about pregnancy.
- Find out the age when the mother and any sisters started their periods, as it may be constitutional. That is, the pulsatile production of GnRH occurs later in some families.
- Determine if there is any family history of any genetic disorders such as Turner's syndrome (if it is mild with only short stature and web neck it may escape notice until puberty).
- Chronic illness, weight loss, anorexia, high levels of exercise or stress can cause hypothalamic dysfunction. Breast milk production might suggest prolactin excess.
- Cyclical abdominal pain may suggest a genitourinary abnormality such as an imperforate hymen or an absent vagina with a functioning uterus.
- Check the past medical history to ensure there is nothing that is likely to have caused amenorrhoea e.g. chemotherapy, as you may not know about previous treatment for a brain tumour, or treatment for a hydrocephalus.

---

**Case study 8.5**

Miss Little attends with her mother who does all the talking. Her mother says she is worried as her daughter, who has just had her 15th birthday, has not yet had a period.

---

## The examination

Check her weight and height to establish her BMI. If the BMI is less than 19, regular menstruation is unlikely. Explain to Miss Little that you need to examine her, but that this will not involve an internal examination. Pelvic examination is not useful or appropriate at this stage. Establish whether she wishes her mother to be present or not – make sure this question is clearly directed to Miss Little, and not to her mother. If you are able to see her alone this gives you another opportunity to check the history (e.g. about risk of pregnancy or anorexia) from her. Chart the secondary sexual characteristics using Table 8.1. You may find it useful to keep a copy of Tanner's stages of puberty in your treatment room for easy access. Look for signs of hypothyroidism, hirsutes, and features of Turner's syndrome. If she consents to you looking at her external genitalia, record your findings.

**Table 8.1:** Tanner's stages of puberty in females[8]

| Stage | Breast | Pubic hair |
| --- | --- | --- |
| 1: Pre-adolescent | Only papillae are elevated. | Vellus hair only, and hair is similar to development over anterior abdominal wall (i.e. no pubic hair). |
| 2 | Breast bud and papilla are elevated and a small mount is present; areola diameter is enlarged. | There is sparse growth of long, slightly pigmented, downy hair or only slightly curled hair, appearing along labia. |
| 3 | Further enlargement of the breast mound; increased palpable glandular tissue. | Hair is darker, coarser, more curled, and spreads to the pubic junction. |
| 4 | Areola and papilla are elevated to form a second mound above the level of the rest of the breast. | Adult-type hair; area covered is less than that in most adults; there is no spread to the medial surface of thighs. |
| 5: Adult | Adult mature breast; recession of areola to the mound of breast tissue, rounding of the breast mound, and projection of only the papillae are evident. | Adult-type hair with increased spread to medial surface of thighs; distribution is as an inverse triangle. |

## Investigations

If she has secondary sexual characteristics and you are at all suspicious, do a pregnancy test. Many young girls deny that they could be pregnant because they have not yet had penetrative sex, although they may have had sexual contact. Some young girls will rule out the possibility of pregnancy because they have not yet started their periods, not recognising that ovulation occurs 14 days before the first menstruation.

Primary amenorrhoea is defined as the failure to establish menstruation by the age of 14 years if there are no signs of secondary sexual maturation, or by the age of

16 years if normal secondary sexual characteristics are developing.[13] Refer for further investigations if a patient falls into either of these categories.

Comprehensive guidance on the management of amenorrhoea in general practice is available from Prodigy.[14]

---

**Case study 8.5 continued**

Miss Little has some secondary sexual characteristics equivalent, you think, to stage 3. Both she and her mother are small and thin and her BMI is only 19. You discuss with her about avoiding smoking and having a good diet. You advise her to increase her calcium intake, how to ensure that she has sufficient sunlight for vitamin D production and to take plenty of weight bearing exercise to maximise her bone mass. You arrange to see her again in six months if she has not started her periods, or before then if any new symptoms appear.

---

## Secondary amenorrhoea

Exclude pregnancy with a pregnancy test. It may seem obvious, but check that she is not receiving a progestogen-only method of contraception (*see* Chapter 5) that would give her irregular periods.

Although it would usually be appropriate to wait until six months of amenorrhoea before initiating other investigations, you decide to commence investigations earlier because of the history of being chronically unwell.

---

**Case study 8.6**

Mrs Reed, a miserable looking thin woman of 39 years, comes to see you because she has not had a proper period for months and is feeling terrible. On enquiry, you eventually determine that her last episode of bleeding was about eight or nine weeks ago, this was particularly heavy, and she has not had a regular cycle for years. She is a frequent visitor to the GP surgery, presenting with multiple somatic complaints.

---

As in primary amenorrhoea, chronic illness or stress can cause hypothalamic dysfunction. Mrs Reed may have problems arising from weight loss or anorexia or possibly high levels of exercise. Enquire about visual field loss as this can occur in a tumour of the pituitary. Breast milk production might suggest prolactin excess. Avoid examining the breasts for expression of milk if you are going to take blood for a prolactin level, as it may raise the level. Ask about symptoms suggestive of thyroid disease. Check that she is not taking any anti-psychotic or other medication that might affect hypothalamic function. Look out for symptoms or signs that would suggest PCOS which occurs in 30% of women with secondary amenorrhoea.[15] Not all patients with PCOS have obesity with hyperpigmentation of the skin folds, but she might have excess body hair, alopecia, acne and a history of difficulty with conception. She might have similar symptoms and signs with rarer conditions like Cushing's syndrome or, if excess body hair has developed rapidly, adrenal hyperplasia, an adrenal tumour or an ovarian androgen-producing tumour.

Symptoms of hot flushes might suggest premature ovarian failure (*see* Chapter 9) and may be associated with autoimmune conditions such as hypothyroidism, diabetes or Addison's disease. Occasionally structural abnormalities of the vagina, stenosis of the cervix or adhesions in the uterus can cause amenorrhoea, usually with complaints of abdominal pain.

## Choosing your investigations

Always do a pregnancy test. Take blood for the levels of FSH, LH, prolactin (*see* Table 8.2 for interpretation in common conditions) and thyroid function in all patients with secondary amenorrhoea. Testosterone levels may be useful in patients with hirsutism. If the levels of testosterone are in the male range, an adrenal or androgenic tumour may be present prompting referral.

Oestradiol blood levels vary too much to be useful, but a progestogen challenge test can show that adequate oestrogens are present. This approach should not be used if you suspect any structural obstruction to the menstrual flow. Medroxyprogesterone acetate 10 mg is given once a day for seven days, and a withdrawal bleed will follow unless oestradiol levels are low.

Pelvic ultrasound may show the classic picture of polycystic ovaries with their 'string of pearls' appearance, from the multiple small peripherally situated cysts.

**Table 8.2:** Hormone results in common causes of amenorrhoea

|  | FSH | LH | Prolactin | Testosterone |
|---|---|---|---|---|
| Hyperprolactaemia (requires further investigation for the cause) | Normal or low | Normal or low | High | Normal |
| PCOS | Normal | Normal or slightly raised | Normal or moderate rise | Slightly raised |
| Premature menopause | Very high | High | Normal | Normal |
| Hypothalamic e.g. with weight loss, excess exercise, stress | Normal or low | Normal or low | Normal | Normal |

When there is doubt about the underlying cause, discuss this with medical colleagues. It is likely that specialist referral may be needed. Patients with a high prolactin will require computerised tomography or magnetic resonance imaging and specialist advice from an endocrinologist.

Correction of underlying causes such as anorexia may require referral to a psychologist or community psychiatric nurse, but lesser degrees of weight loss or over-exercising can be successfully managed in primary care with regular support and consistent advice.

PCOS responds best to weight loss.[16] Patients often require treatment for associated lipid disorders, diabetes or hypertension.[17] Treatment with metformin is sometimes given but evidence for prevention of long-term adverse outcomes is not yet available.

---

**Case study 8.6 continued**

Mrs Reed's investigations are all normal except for a slightly raised prolactin level. You tell her that her tests do not suggest that she is menopausal as she assumed. You suggest that she keeps a record of her menstrual loss over the next six months.

---

# Postcoital bleeding

You need to establish whether Miss Angst feels she is at risk of having *Chlamydia*, which is a common cause of intermenstrual bleeding. Ask whether there has been a change of sexual partner in the past six months and make Miss Angst aware of the incidence of *Chlamydia*. The information that the bleeding is mainly postcoital helps with the possible diagnosis. The most likely causes are cervical ectopy, polyps, infection or malignancy. Cervical ectopy is more common while taking the contraceptive pill, so this is the most likely cause. A vaginal examination using a speculum to inspect the cervix will show whether an ectopy is present and you can then tell the patient about this condition.

---

**Case study 8.7**

Miss Angst visits you for a repeat prescription of the combined pill. Although she is happy with the method, she tells you that she is concerned because she has occasional intermenstrual bleeding, and sometimes bleeds after intercourse.

---

Although it is often called cervical ectopy or cervical erosion, the correct term is cervical ectropion. Ectropion is defined as 'a rolling outward of the margin of a part'. Cervical erosion acquired its name from the appearance of the cervix as the deeper pinky-red area around the cervical os looks as though some of the surface has come off, but is due to the columnar epithelium from the cervical canal moving out (almost like a flower opening) to cover part of the vaginal cervix. Ectropion is normal for many women at some time in their menstrual cycle, but is more common with higher levels of oestrogen in pregnancy or while taking combined contraceptive hormones. Some pills are more likely to affect the condition than others, so Miss Angst may want to change to one with less oestrogen, or with a higher level of progestogen. She may want to change to a method without oestrogen (*see* Chapter 5). If it persists, or if she has a lot of vaginal discharge associated with it, there are surgical procedures for dealing with this issue, almost all of them the ones used for the treatment of pre-invasive cervical disease (dysplasia), such as freezing (cryotherapy) or heat treatment (diathermy). They are generally effective, but there is a very small risk of infertility. It is important to tell Miss Angst that this is not a condition associated with infection, nor does it increase her risk of cancer.

Cervical visualisation will also reveal any cervicitis. While undertaking vaginal examination, it would be useful to also take endo-cervical swabs to test for *Chlamydia*, providing the patient understands your reasons for doing this and has given her informed consent (*see* Chapter 6).

If she has not had a recent cervical smear, you might consider doing a diagnostic cervical smear, marking on the form your reasons for the investigation.

It may be difficult to decide from the history if her problem is mainly intermenstrual bleeding that sometimes also occurs after intercourse or is mainly postcoital bleeding. Keeping a daily record of any bleeding may help to sort this out. A record can also help if Miss Angst has been forgetting to take her contraceptive pills, or taking them at irregular times so that hormonal fluctuations may be triggering a withdrawal loss.

If Miss Angst continues to have postcoital bleeding and has no obvious cause, or if she has an unusual-looking cervix, arrange for her referral for colposcopy. If she is over 40 years of age, and continues to have bleeding even after stopping hormonal contraception, she might also need examination of the endometrium by endometrial sampling, transvaginal scan or hysteroscopy.

# Collecting data to demonstrate your learning, competence, performance and standards of service delivery

## Example cycle of evidence 8.1

- Focus: clinical care
- Other relevant focus: maintaining good medical practice

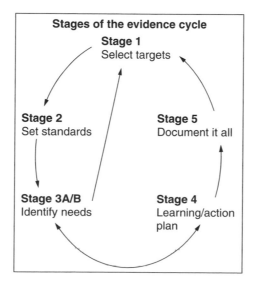

**Stages of the evidence cycle**

**Stage 1**
Select targets

**Stage 2**
Set standards

**Stage 5**
Document it all

**Stage 3A/B**
Identify needs

**Stage 4**
Learning/action plan

---

**Case study 8.8**

Mrs Razor presents at a well woman clinic, troubled that her periods have become irregular. She is unhappy with her body image and she wishes to lose weight, which has been gradually increasing since her 40th birthday last year. She now weighs 90 kg at a height of 1.65 m. As you discuss her problems, it becomes apparent that something is causing her worry and embarrassment. Eventually she summons the courage to tell you that her main problem is that she has more frequently needed to shave her legs, and she is worried that she is becoming more 'hairy'.

---

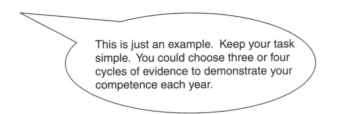

This is just an example. Keep your task simple. You could choose three or four cycles of evidence to demonstrate your competence each year.

## *Stage 1: Select your aspirations for good practice*

The excellent nurse:

- is sympathetic to the concerns of patients and recognises the presenting complaint may not always be the main concern
- provides patients with the opportunity and the confidence to discuss sensitive issues.

## *Stage 2: Set the standards for your outcomes*

Outcomes might include:

- the way learning is applied
- a learnt skill
- a protocol
- a strategy that is implemented
- meeting recommended standards.

- Demonstrate that you address weight problems for patients who consult with obesity.
- Demonstrate consistent best practice in the recognition and management of PCOS and related problems.

*Stage 3A: Identify your learning needs*

- Self-assess and reflect on your own learning needs in respect of PCOS with regard to diagnosis and management.
- Carry out a significant event audit of delayed diagnosis in cases of PCOS.

*Stage 3B: Identify your service needs*

> Any of the needs assessment exercises in 3A may also reveal service needs.

- Review the advice provided in your practice to obese individuals who wish to lose weight – how does it compare against national guidelines? Establish whether patients are contacted when they default from weight loss programmes.
- Audit the records of patients with important co-morbidities such as diabetes mellitus and hypertension, to see if appropriate advice about diet and weight has been given.

*Stage 4: Make and carry out a learning and action plan*

- Visit the local nursing library and search for recent articles on PCOS to update your knowledge.
- Arrange an informal presentation (from yourself or an invited speaker) for your colleagues to discuss the implications and management of obesity and PCOS.
- Create or find a patient information leaflet about PCOS.[18]
- Discuss at a team meeting how a system of contacting patients who default from weight loss programmes might be established to make them feel that the practice was concerned and keen to help.
- Visit the dietician to discuss how you can improve the advice and support you offer to patients with obesity.

*Stage 5: Document your learning, competence, performance and standards of service delivery*

- Write your own notes about the recognition and management of PCOS, and keep a record of key references including useful website pages to use in teaching colleagues, and to keep in your portfolio.
- Record in your reflective diary the comments from patients (suitably anonymised) who are contacted when they default from weight loss programmes.
- Record the changes to the advice and support you offer to patients with obesity.

---

**Case study 8.8 continued**

Following confirmation of the diagnosis of PCOS by ultrasound scan and slight elevation of serum androgens, Mrs Razor was relieved to hear the explanation of her symptoms. Recognising the importance of weight reduction, Mrs Razor has altered her lifestyle to increase the amount of exercise taken and is aiming for gradual but sustained weight reduction with a dietary plan. She visits you for a weekly weight check to maintain her motivation.

---

# Example cycle of evidence 8.2

- Focus: relationship with patients

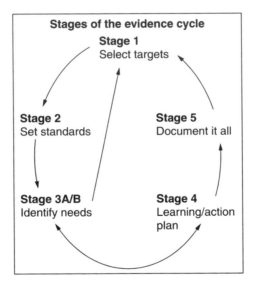

---

**Case study 8.9**

Miss Fret is a 23 year old who attends for a repeat cervical smear. She tells you that she is concerned because her previous smear result was reported as 'abnormal'. She remembers the nurse who took the smear telling her that she had an erosion and she is now worrying that her cervix is being eaten away with cervical cancer and wonders if this is because she has been taking 'the pill' for more than five years. She tells you that she occasionally experiences a blood-stained discharge, and this is often worse after sexual intercourse has occurred.

---

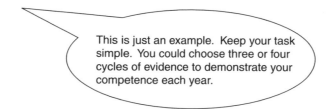

This is just an example. Keep your task simple. You could choose three or four cycles of evidence to demonstrate your competence each year.

## Stage 1: Select your aspirations for good practice

The excellent nurse will:

- listen to patients' concerns
- be aware when symptoms necessitate referral and when reassurance can safely be given
- dispel myths that have no evidence base.

## Stage 2: Set the standards for your outcomes

Outcomes might include:

- the way learning is applied
- a learnt skill
- a protocol
- a strategy that is implemented
- meeting recommended standards.

- Establishment of appropriate patient education for people with 'abnormal' cervical smear reports.
- A patient education leaflet for information about cervical ectopy.

## Stage 3A: Identify your learning needs

- Consider what you know and what patients should know about cervical ectopy and postcoital bleeding.
- Review the information given to patients with cervical ectopy.

## Stage 3B: Identify your service needs

Any of the needs assessment exercises in 3A may also reveal service needs.

- Review the quality of information given to patients by yourself and others about cervical smears and vaginal blood loss.

- Find out the latest figures on the availability and accessibility of investigations and treatment for cancers of the cervix.

### Stage 4: Make and carry out a learning and action plan

- Discuss with colleagues what information is given to patients who are noted to have cervical ectopy on examination. Rehearse ways of explaining this occurrence using language that is understandable and not emotive.
- Review how information is given to patients when their smear result is abnormal or needs repeating for any reason. Write a variety of sample letters and circulate them amongst female staff, including the cleaners, to determine the least worrying way of asking patients to return for a repeat smear.
- Ask patients for feedback about the information they received and record this in your reflective diary.

### Stage 5: Document your learning, competence, performance and standards of service delivery

- Create a patient leaflet that explains what is meant by cervical ectopy and gives details of the possible symptoms. Include this in your portfolio to demonstrate how you have responded to anxious patients in a positive manner.
- Include the feedback from patients about the information they received.
- Include the results of the availability and accessibility of investigations and treatment for cancers of the cervix and that you have passed these onto the practice manager for action about the deficiencies identified.

---

**Case study 8.9 continued**

Six weeks later, Miss Fret returns to see you for a repeat prescription of the pill. You are able to give her the smear results, which are negative. She tells you that the occasional blood-stained discharge is still present but she is no longer concerned because she understands why it occurs. You remind her to return if she experiences any worsening of symptoms.

---

# Example cycle of evidence 8.3

- Focus: working with colleagues
- Other relevant focus: teaching and training

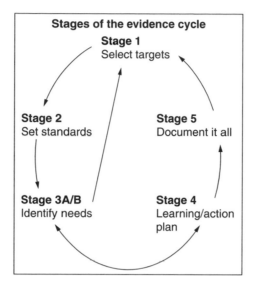

**Stages of the evidence cycle**

**Stage 1**
Select targets

**Stage 2**
Set standards

**Stage 5**
Document it all

**Stage 3A/B**
Identify needs

**Stage 4**
Learning/action plan

---

**Case study 8.10**

The local clinical nurse specialist notes your interest in early pregnancy loss after you request to attend her clinic as an observer. She offers to help you draw up guidelines for the management of patients who have recurrent miscarriages.

---

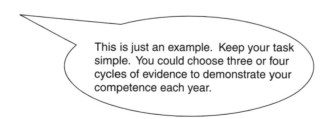

This is just an example. Keep your task simple. You could choose three or four cycles of evidence to demonstrate your competence each year.

## Stage 1: Select your aspirations for good practice

The excellent nurse:

- respects the views of colleagues and patients when developing group guidelines on best practice
- helps to train professional colleagues and share knowledge.

*Stage 2: Set the standards for your outcomes*

Outcomes might include:

- the way learning is applied
- a learnt skill
- a protocol
- a strategy that is implemented
- meeting recommended standards.

- Develop practice guidelines for management of recurrent miscarriage including availability of local resources and best practice from national guidelines.
- The guidelines include a specific nursing focus to develop the role of psychological support and to highlight the need to recognise the loss as significant.

*Stage 3A: Identify your learning needs*

- Arrange to visit your local pregnancy assessment unit and ask the midwives to direct you to the most recent literature on recurrent miscarriage.
- Ask what tests should be undertaken for women presenting with miscarriage. Find out the purpose of the tests so that you can inform women about these from an educated perspective.

*Stage 3B: Identify your service needs*

Any of the needs assessment exercises in 3A may also reveal service needs.

- Assess current practice: review the investigations undertaken in the primary care setting for the last three patients presenting with recurrent miscarriage.

*Stage 4: Make and carry out a learning and action plan*

- Find out what services are available locally for women who miscarry. This should include the provision of counselling services and voluntary organisations.
- Discuss the current management with colleagues and then agree how your standards could be improved.

*Stage 5: Document your learning, competence, performance and standards of service delivery*

- Keep a copy in your portfolio of the guidelines you have produced, with a short rationale that explains how they were created.
- Create a resource file of contact names/numbers of local organisations who offer support after miscarriage.

---

**Case study 8.10 continued**

You find that drafting guidelines for your practice or the local area is a good educational process that raises interest in the topic and encourages working effectively with your colleagues.

---

# References

1   www.rcog.org.uk/guidelines.asp?PageID=108&GuidelineID=28

2   Vessey M, Villard L, Mackintosh M *et al.* (1992) The epidemiology of hysterectomy: findings in a large cohort study. *British Journal of Obstetrics and Gynaecology.* **99**: 402–7.

3   Porteous A and Prentice A (2003) Medical management of dysfunctional uterine bleeding. *Reviews in Gynaecological Practice.* **3**: 81–4.

4   Lethaby A, Cooke I and Rees M (2002) Progesterone/progestogen releasing intrauterine system for heavy menstrual bleeding (Cochrane Review). *The Cochrane Library, Issue 4, 2002.* Update Software, Oxford.

5   Barrington JW and Bowen-Simpkins P (1997) The levonorgestrel intrauterine system in the management of menorrhagia. *British Journal of Obstetrics and Gynaecology.* **104**: 614–16.

6   Sowter MC (2003) New surgical treatments for menorrhagia. *Lancet.* **361**: 1456–8.

7   Pron G, Bennett J, Common A *et al.* and Ontario Uterine Fibroid Embolization Collaborative Group (2003) The Ontario Uterine Fibroid Embolization Trial. Part 2. Uterine fibroid reduction and symptom relief after uterine artery embolization for fibroids. *Fertility and Sterility.* **79**: 120–7.

8   Sagsveen M, Farmer JE, Prentice A and Breeze A (2004) Gonadotrophin-releasing hormone analogues for endometriosis: bone mineral density (Cochrane Review). *The Cochrane Library, Issue 2, 2004.* John Wiley and Sons Ltd, Chichester.

9   Winkel CA (2003) Evaluation and management of women with endometriosis. *Obstetrics and Gynecology.* **102**: 397–408.

10   www.rcog.org.uk/guidelines.asp?PageID=106&GuidelineID=10

11   www.rcog.org.uk/guidelines.asp?PageID=106&GuidelinesID=8

12   www.miscarriageassociation.org.uk or www.babyloss.com

13   Marshall WA and Tanner JM (1969) Variations in pattern of pubertal changes in girls. *Archives of Disease in Childhood.* **44(235)**: 291–303.

14   www.prodigy.nhs.uk/guidance.asp?gt=Amenorrhoea

15   Edmonds DK (ed.) (1999) *Dewhurst's Textbook of Obstetrics and Gynaecology for Post-graduates* (6e). Blackwell Science, Oxford.

16   Andrews G (2001) *Women's Sexual Health* (2e). Baillière Tindall, London.

17   Harris C and Carey A (2000) *A Woman's Guide to Dealing with Polycystic Ovary Syndrome.* Thorsons, London.

18   www.pcos-support.org/

# 9

# The menopause

---

**Case study 9.1**

A 46-year-old woman comes to see you with irregular periods and asks if she could be 'on the change'.

---

# What issues you should cover

## Age

Usually the menopause happens between the ages of 48 and 54 years, but it may occur outside these ages. The median age of menopause is 51 years old. The *menopause* is the permanent stopping of menstruation resulting from loss of ovarian follicle activity. The natural menopause is defined as being after 12 months of no menstruation, so can only be decided after the event.

The *perimenopause* includes the time beginning with the first features of the approaching menopause, such as hot flushes or menstrual irregularity. It ends 12 months after the last menstrual period. The *postmenopause* starts with the last menstrual period but cannot be dated with certainty until 12 months have occurred without menstruation.

A *premature menopause* is usually defined as the permanent cessation of menstrual periods due to loss of ovarian follicular activity occurring before 40 years of age. A *surgical menopause* occurs when the ovaries are removed. This is sometimes done together with a hysterectomy and causes a sudden drop in female hormone level, often with severe symptoms.

## Timing of her last period

She could be having menopausal symptoms even if she is still having menstrual periods (perimenopause) but you would also want to think about alternative reasons for hot sweats (e.g. anxiety, pyrexia) or psychological symptoms (e.g. worsening premenstrual syndrome or depression).[1]

If she has not had a recent period, ensure that she is not pregnant. Many women think that they cannot become pregnant if they are coming up to 50 years of age and stop using contraception. If she is at risk of pregnancy, arrange a pregnancy test and discuss contraceptive precautions with her.[2,3]

If she has been having periods, she may be worried because she has missed periods or had them more frequently and that the amount of loss is different. Periods may become closer together when ovulation is not occurring because the luteal phase is shortened. The luteal phase occurs after ovulation when the corpus luteum, formed from the cells around the released ovum, produces progesterone to maintain the endometrium ready for a fertilised ovum. Irregular loss of the endometrium occurs when insufficient progesterone is produced. This loss is light or absent if oestrogen levels are also lowered. The loss can be heavy if oestrogen levels are fluctuating and are sometimes high enough to increase the thickness of the endometrium.

## Hot flushes

If she has been having hot flushes, establish how often they are occurring, how much of a nuisance they are and whether they are disturbing her sleep. Being woken several times a night can lead to irritability and loss of concentration the following day, especially if she has to get out of bed to change nightwear or sheets because of sweating.

## Vaginal dryness

Thinning of the vaginal walls, less lubrication, and discomfort with sexual intercourse tend to occur after several years of lowered hormone levels but some women will develop this earlier. Use direct questions, as many women will not volunteer this information but will be grateful for a chance to discuss it.

## Formication

You may also need to ask about this condition of feeling as if something is crawling just under the skin, as many women do not like to mention it. They often think that it is a sign of a psychiatric illness and are very reassured to discover that it can occur as a symptom of the menopause.

## Bladder symptoms

Urgency and frequency of micturition are often associated with vaginal dryness and she may have noticed a tendency to have more frequent urinary tract infections. Incontinence or difficulties passing urine are more likely to be associated with structural abnormalities such as urogenital prolapse.

## Psychological symptoms

Contrary to popular belief, there is no clear evidence that changes in hormone levels at the menopause can cause depression. Most women do not have major mood changes around their menopause and those that do usually have other reasons for their symptoms.[4–6] The physical changes of the menopause may make it more difficult to cope with the many major life stresses that occur in 40–60 year olds of both sexes. If psychological symptoms are prominent, enquire about other stressful events such as:

- parents ageing and becoming dependent
- deaths of family or friends
- loss of partner through death, separation or divorce
- children leaving home
- demanding workload
- family worries such as partner's job, children's marriages, etc
- poor health
- money worries
- coming to terms with her own ageing.

## Worries about osteoporosis[7,8]

If she is concerned about having thinning of her bones, establish if this is because she has symptoms of aching or swelling of her joints. Symptoms will need independent evaluation for their cause but are often part of the ageing process rather than being due to menopausal changes.

A family history such as a mother or sister with osteoporosis is associated with a higher risk of developing it herself. Other factors that might give her a higher risk are:

- an established menopause before the age of 45 years
- being underweight
- smoking
- taking little physical exercise
- treatment with corticosteroids
- a poor diet with little calcium or vitamin D intake
- excess alcohol intake
- a fragility fracture (one occurring with minimal trauma such as slipping over)
- having a medical condition such as rheumatoid arthritis, malabsorption syndromes (Crohn's disease, ulcerative colitis, gluten sensitivity), liver or parathyroid disease.

## Reasons for hormonal blood test

Many women ask if they can have a blood test to determine whether they are 'on the change'. If a woman has already stopped having periods, there is little point unless she requires investigation because she might have a premature menopause. The variable level of hormones in people having periods makes hormonal blood tests largely irrelevant too (see Box 9.1). The only indication for blood tests is if the history is suggestive of a condition other than a straightforward menopausal transition.

---

**Box 9.1:**   Blood tests for menopausal symptoms

*Follicle stimulating hormone* (FSH) is only helpful if the level is in the menopausal range (over 30 IU/l). The level fluctuates widely when a woman is still having menstrual loss and is going through the perimenopause. The level is controlled by the pulsatile release of GnRH from the hypothalamus, and is affected by feedback from oestrogen and progesterone levels as well as by inhibin. Several measurements over a period of time may be required if a premature menopause is suspected.

*Oestradiol* levels are not useful in the diagnosis of the menopause, either premature or at the usual time, because of the variation in levels from day to day and even at various times of day. Oestradiol levels can be used to check the levels of circulating hormone before replacement of subcutaneous implants of oestrogen, or to check levels absorbed from the skin or mucus membranes. Oestrogen given orally is mainly converted to oestrone so that oestradiol levels are not helpful.

*Thyroid function tests* may be useful when doubt arises as to whether symptoms are actually menopausal. Tiredness, weight gain, hair loss and flushes may indicate an underactive thyroid rather than ovarian failure.

---

# What she may know about the menopause

She may say that she has read lots about it and has come to you to find out more about hormone replacement therapy (HRT). A nursing consultation should focus on patient education including what the patient can do herself to combat the effects of the menopause.[9] She may want to discuss:

- identifying the things that trigger the flushes, e.g. hot drinks, caffeine, spicy food, alcohol, and reducing or avoiding them
- wearing layers of clothing so that some can be removed easily when she has a flush
- relaxation techniques to avoid feeling stressed and rushed, as anxiety can make flushes more frequent
- taking regular exercise, eating healthily and avoiding smoking
- using lubricants to make sexual intercourse more comfortable
- using plant substances that have similar effects to those of oestrogens.[10] There is some evidence that phytoestrogens might be helpful. The two important groups of foods containing phytoestrogens are: isoflavones that are found in soybeans, chick peas, red clover and probably other legumes; and lignans that are found in linseeds and smaller amounts in cereal bran, vegetables, legumes and fruit. However, phytoestrogens are unlikely to have a major effect on symptoms[11]
- using other alternative therapies, e.g. acupuncture or homeopathy although little firm evidence exists that they are helpful.[12,13]

Be cautious about the claims for other herbal treatments, some of which may interact with prescribed medications (e.g. warfarin, antidepressants). Others may contain toxic chemicals such as pesticides, mercury, arsenic and lead. Black cohosh has been approved in Germany for treatment of the menopause, and St John's Wort can help with mild depressive symptoms.

Progesterone cream is sold for treatment of menopausal symptoms. Insufficient is absorbed to be bone-protective, or to provide protection for the endometrium if oestrogen replacement therapy is used, but some women report lessening of symptom severity.

## Advising on hormone replacement therapy (HRT)

If you have had a long consultation already, you might at this stage give the woman some information on HRT to take away with her. Establishing a small patient library with books,[14] videos and leaflets relating to the menopause will be helpful and informative for patients. Ensure that the information is as up to date as you can find because of the rapidly changing information available. She can return to see you better informed and better able to discuss the advantages and disadvantages of treatment.

The consensus opinion in the UK is that HRT should be used for symptom relief, at the lowest dose and for the shortest time compatible with the control of unacceptable symptoms.[15–17] You will need to find out the opinions of the medical colleagues with whom you work. Many health professionals are poorly informed about the risks and benefits of HRT and may have biased opinions based on incomplete or inaccurate information. You need to be able to refer to those who are able and willing to discuss the options from evidence-based information. Some conditions that have received publicity recently may need specific discussion, and you should be aware of the conclusions from the studies and their limitations. HRT should not be recommended when there is an increased risk of the following conditions, or for the prevention of these conditions:[17,18]

- *cardiovascular disease:* the risk of heart attacks and strokes is slightly increased, mainly in the first couple of years of use
- *venous thromboembolism:* there is a 2–3-fold increase in risk with oral preparations. This may not apply to transdermal therapy. The background risk of thrombosis in menopausal women is about 1 in 10 000 women per year. Using HRT will increase this by about two to four extra women in every 10 000 developing a thrombosis each year
- *endometrial cancer:* oestrogen-only and sequential combined HRT appear to increase the risk slightly, but continuous combined therapy appears to be slightly protective
- *breast cancer:* the excess risk of breast cancer appears to be similar to that attributable to a late menopause. Although small in absolute terms, it has provoked much alarm. Combined therapy was found in recent studies to give the greatest risk (an additional six per thousand cases after five years of use), oestrogen-only therapy giving only a very small extra risk (an additional 1.5 per thousand cases after five years of use), and tibolone (*see* Box 9.3) an intermediate risk. In women aged 50–64 years, the baseline risk is 32 per thousand, so this increases the risk to 33.5 per thousand for those taking oestrogen-only therapy and 38 per thousand for combined therapy users. Five years after stopping HRT, the woman's risk of breast cancer is the same as for women who have never taken it. If women are taking HRT at the time their breast cancer is diagnosed, their life expectancy does

not seem to be reduced. It is not known if this is because cancers are diagnosed at an earlier stage in HRT users, or because the HRT has an effect on the cancer.[17–21]

The previous suggestion that HRT might protect against Alzheimer's disease has not been confirmed, although the greater risk of dementia might be due to the pro-thrombotic effects of HRT.

HRT is protective against osteoporosis and prevents fractures. However, other therapies, such as biphosphonates, should be considered if there are no other indications for HRT, if lifestyle changes and calcium and vitamin D supplements are insufficient.

Most other conditions appear to be unaffected by HRT although colorectal cancer incidence appears to be reduced.

If the woman is already well informed and the consultation has been short you might continue. Take a history for conditions that might be affected by HRT. Physical examination should include measurement of her blood pressure and BMI. The Royal College of Nursing advises against nurses undertaking breast examination because of the risk of giving false reassurance to women. However, encourage breast awareness so that women spot any early changes in appearance. Mammography has a higher sensitivity and specificity for breast cancer than clinical examination. Participation in national screening programmes should be encouraged. Nurses should familiarise themselves with local arrangements for mammography so that they can discuss when invitations are likely to arrive and explain what is involved. Women should also be encouraged to participate in the cervical screening programme. You will need to know more about her irregular periods. If she has heavy irregular periods that are more frequent, or if she has intermenstrual bleeding, investigation of the cause would be indicated before the use of HRT.

HRT consists of an oestrogen, which may be combined with a progestogen in women who have not had a hysterectomy. The hormone(s) can be absorbed by different routes: oral, transdermal, subcutaneous, intranasal and vaginal. Most women will now be started on 1 mg oestradiol orally, 50 µg transdermally, or 25 mg implanted oestradiol, unless the woman has a premature menopause or also has severe osteoporosis.

Women may be given an oestrogen subcutaneous implant after a total hysterectomy and bilateral oophorectomy but this method of administration can be difficult to manage (*see* Box 9.2).

---

**Box 9.2:**   Management of oestrogen implants

Use of subcutaneous implants was associated with tachyphylaxis i.e. menopausal symptoms returned and a further implant was given even while the blood levels of oestradiol were high. Very high levels of oestradiol could be attained after repeated implants. Although the risk of this occurring appeared low, some women were intolerant of symptoms and demanded early replacement of the implant. The management now advised is not to replace an implant until oestradiol levels are no higher than 400 pmol/l.[22]

Tibolone is a synthetic hormone that has mixed oestrogenic, progestogenic and androgenic actions, and is used by women who do not want to have bleeding (*see* Box 9.3).

---

**Box 9.3:**   How tibolone differs from oestrogen plus progestogen replacement therapy

- Like oestrogen, it alleviates menopausal symptoms but its effect on the endometrium is like that of progestogen. Cyclical bleeding is not promoted.
- Vaginal cell maturation is normalised and symptomatic atrophic vaginitis is relieved with reduction in vaginal dryness and dyspareunia.
- Randomised studies have shown improvements in mood compared with placebo, and similar effects on adverse mood to conventional HRT.
- It significantly reduces sex hormone binding globulin and has some androgenic effects. Improvements in sexual functioning are greater than those seen with conventional HRT.
- It has oestrogenic effects on bone density.
- Tibolone inhibits proliferation of human breast cells. The incidence of breast tenderness is low and breast density is not increased unlike with conventional HRT. It is not known if this translates into clinical significance for the risk of breast cancer.
- No increase in thrombotic events in women taking tibolone has been reported in the literature (but this may be due to the small numbers of women taking it).

Tibolone does not suit every woman and may provide inadequate relief of symptoms in some women. Some complain of progestogen-like side-effects.[23]

---

## Starting HRT

If menstruation has not stopped, a GP or specialist is likely to have started HRT with a monthly (or three-monthly) sequential cyclical preparation to try to promote a regular bleeding pattern. Once no menstruation has occurred for 12 months, a continuous combined, no bleed, preparation can be tried. Even if you are not a nurse prescriber, patients will expect you to have some knowledge of HRT. Nurses who accept responsibility for medication management in chronic conditions can make an enormous difference to improving compliance rates. It is sensible to become familiar with a few of the large range of HRT therapies available, rather than attempting to know about all the preparations in detail. Talking to the doctors you work with about the particular preparations they are most likely to prescribe, and why, will be useful. It can help you to draw up a list of therapies that patients are most likely to ask about and doctors should be able to give you the rationale for prescribing in a particular manner. The cost of the preparation must feature in the decision-making process of what to prescribe, but equally important is determining the acceptability to the woman. After discussing the advantages and disadvantages of HRT, doctors frequently refer patients on to nurses in order to provide an opportunity for patients to look at the full range of delivery systems. Oral medication is generally cheaper than other options, but the woman should have an opportunity to discuss exactly what she would prefer. If you build up a supply of placebo options that patients can handle, it will help women to decide which type they would prefer to use.

## Switching from sequential to continuous combined therapy

When women are postmenopausal and still require HRT for symptom control, they should be switched from sequential to continuous combined preparations. By the age of 54 years, 80% of women are postmenopausal. Most women who have had six months without any bleeding, or who have had raised FSH levels after the mid-40s, are postmenopausal.

## Protecting the endometrium in women who have not had a hysterectomy

Progestogens are added to reduce the risk of hyperplasia and carcinoma of the endometrium that occurs with unopposed oestrogen. Women who have had endometrial ablation need progestogens, as it cannot be assumed that all the endometrium has been removed. Standard sequential or continuous combined therapy contain suitable levels of progestogen to protect the endometrium. Although not licensed yet in the UK for this indication, a Mirena intrauterine system can be used to provide both contraception and endometrial protection and can be particularly useful if the woman has unacceptable progestogenic side-effects such as bloating, acne or premenstrual syndrome symptoms.[24] Changing the progestogen to dydrogesterone may also reduce progestogenic side-effects. Most women who have had a hysterectomy can take oestrogen alone.

## Treatment of urogenital symptoms

These are best treated with vaginally administered low-dose natural oestrogens, such as oestriol by cream or pessary, or oestradiol by tablet or from a ring. Nurses may encounter women with atrophic vaginitis when taking routine cervical smears. This provides a perfect opportunity to raise the issue of urogenital symptoms or dyspareunia. Long-term treatment with local oestrogen is needed or symptoms will recur. With the recommended dosage regimes, no endometrial effects should occur and it is not necessary to add a progestogen.

## How long should HRT be continued?[25]

- *Treatment of flushes and other symptoms:* continue while symptoms affect the quality of life, but re-evaluate benefits and risks after symptoms have resolved, and have a trial without HRT.
- *Prevention or treatment of osteoporosis:* HRT would have to be continued for life as bone mineral density falls once treatment is stopped. Most women and their health

professionals will choose to transfer to other bone-protective agents once menopausal symptoms have stopped.
* *Premature menopause:* continue until at least the median age of menopause (51 years), then re-evaluate benefits and risks.

# Non-oestrogen treatments

After discussion about the benefits and risks of HRT you may advise against HRT or the woman may decide against it. Other medication should then be considered if she has risk factors.

## *Osteoporosis*

If the main indication for treatment is prevention or treatment of osteoporosis then other medication may be preferable (*see* Table 9.1 and Box 9.4) and women should be encouraged to ask their GP about whether these may be appropriate (or they may wish you to ask on their behalf).

**Table 9.1:** Prevention and treatment of osteoporosis. Royal College of Physicians' grade of recommendations for therapy[7]

| Treatment | Spine | Hip |
|---|---|---|
| Etridronate | A | B |
| Aledronate | A | A |
| Risedronate | A | A |
| Calcium and vitamin D | ND | A |
| Calcium | A | B |
| Calcitriol | A | ND |
| Calcitonin | A | B |
| Selective oestrogen receptor modulators (*see* Box 9.4) | A | ND |

A = good evidence from randomly controlled trials.

B = evidence from observational or case controlled trials.

ND = not demonstrated.

---

**Box 9.4:** Selective oestrogen receptor modulators (SERMs)[23]

This class of compounds act as oestrogens in some locations and anti-oestrogens in others. Tamoxifen, the first SERM, is widely used as a treatment for breast cancer containing oestrogen receptors. Its use is associated with a raised risk of venous thrombosis and of endometrial cancer.

Raloxifene, the second SERM to be commercially available, has shown a good reduction of the risk of breast cancer in people receiving it for prevention of osteoporosis. The coronary heart risk was also reduced. Further long-term studies are needed to confirm these findings.

> SERMs increase hot flushes and the risk of venous thrombosis. Trials are underway to determine if a combination of a low-dose oestradiol with a SERM might improve the risk profile. This would relieve hot flushes, protect the breast and bone mass and, it is hoped, have a neutral effect on the endometrium.

## Hot flushes and other symptoms[26]

Progestogens can be helpful, e.g. norethisterone 5 mg/day or megestrol acetate 40 mg/day. Clonidine has also been shown to reduce flushing but this research was based on one trial when it was used transdermally. This formulation is not currently available in the UK. Early results from trials suggest that selective serotonin re-uptake inhibitors (SSRIs) e.g. venlafaxine/paroxetine may be helpful although they are not yet licensed for this indication.

## Vaginal atrophy

Recommend vaginal lubricants to purchase, together with discussion about why vaginal dryness is occurring, and reassurance that this does not mean that women should refrain from a regular sex life. Become familiar with the lubricants available in pharmacies, shops and on the Internet.

# When to refer[25]

Nurses in primary care who are well educated in effects of the menopause and HRT can manage the care of most women taking HRT. However, the following conditions warrant prompt medical referral, and will frequently require specialist intervention:

- *abnormal bleeding:*
  - before starting HRT – a sudden change in menstrual pattern, intermenstrual bleeding, postcoital bleeding or a postmenopausal bleed
  - sequential HRT – a change in the pattern of withdrawal bleed or breakthrough bleeding (BTB)
  - continuous combined HRT – BTB for more than 4–6 months after starting or that is not lessening. Bleeding after complete amenorrhoea
- *multiple treatment failures:* after more than three types of HRT preparations have been tried. List what has been given and the problems encountered
- *confirmed venous thrombosis:* either in the patient's personal history or in a first-degree relative under the age of 50 years
- *premature menopause:* to determine the reason for the menopause under 40 years of age
- *osteoporosis risk:* to help with the assessment for the treatment dose required and the response to treatment (refer for bone mineral density scans if available in your area)
- *previous or high risk of hormone dependent cancer:* e.g. breast, ovarian, endometrial cancer.

You might wish to join a professional organisation such as the British Menopause Society so that you keep up to date with a rapidly changing field. [27]

# Collecting data to demonstrate your learning, competence, performance and standards of service delivery

## Example cycle of evidence 9.1

- Focus: clinical care
- Other relevant focus: working with colleagues

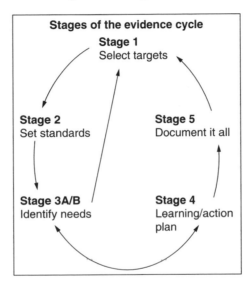

**Stages of the evidence cycle**

**Stage 1**
Select targets

**Stage 2**
Set standards

**Stage 5**
Document it all

**Stage 3A/B**
Identify needs

**Stage 4**
Learning/action plan

---

**Case study 9.2**

Mrs Muddle is 55 years old. She comes to see you to have a routine smear performed. Her medical notes show that she recently visited her GP with symptoms of urinary frequency, dysuria and 'soreness down below'. A MSU sample had been sent off, but this showed no sign of infection. The result had been marked with a 'no action' stamp. You ask if she still has symptoms and find that she does. The labelling of the MSU as 'normal' had prevented Mrs Muddle from attending again as she thought this meant she had to put up with her symptoms. You want to prevent a recurrence of this situation with other patients.

---

This is just an example. Keep your task simple. You could choose three or four cycles of evidence to demonstrate your competence each year.

## Stage 1: Select your aspirations for good practice

The excellent nurse:

- makes an adequate assessment of the patient's condition, based on the history and, if indicated, an appropriate examination
- provides or arrange investigations or treatment where necessary
- keeps clear, legible and contemporaneous records that include clinical findings, decisions made, information given to patients and any treatments given or prescribed.

## Stage 2: Set the standards for your outcomes

Outcomes might include:

- the way learning is applied
- a learnt skill
- a protocol
- a strategy that is implemented
- meeting recommended standards.

- Demonstrate consistent best practice in assessment and treatment of postmeno-pausal urogenital atrophy.
- Demonstrate best practice in consistency of approach through teamwork.

## Stage 3A: Identify your learning needs

- Determine what barriers to best practice exist by a record review of 10 other patients who present to yourself and other colleagues with similar symptoms.
- Review how results are interpreted and relayed to patients.

## Stage 3B: Identify your service needs

Any of the needs assessment exercises in 3A may also reveal service needs.

- Track what happens to MSU reports when received by the practice.
- Discuss with other health professionals their response to MSU results that are reported as 'negative' or 'white blood cells and no growth' and what they record that the patient should be told.
- Discuss with the team (including reception staff) what information is given to patients about their MSU results from the comments written on the report by the health professional.

- Undertake a SWOT analysis of the way records are made and kept (storage, paper-based, electronic, coding etc) with others in the practice team.

## Stage 4: Make and carry out a learning and action plan

- Read about urogenital atrophy, its symptoms and treatment.
- Write up the record review (that shows perhaps that most women are being treated in accordance with best practice, but that a few women with urinary symptoms of urogenital atrophy are not having a discussion of treatment options).
- Discuss the record review with other health professionals and agree to change the wording of the instructions to the practice staff from 'no infection' to 'no infection, please see the doctor if you still have symptoms' to provide a fail-safe mechanism.
- Create a protocol for discussion with the team to highlight the best treatment options for urogenital atrophy.

## Stage 5: Document your learning, competence, performance and standards of service delivery

- Use a reminder on the practice audit calendar and repeat the record review in six months to confirm that the changes are working.
- Document the discussion of your results with other health professionals and obtain their feedback.
- Obtain feedback from practice staff about interactions with patients over the giving of MSU results.
- Keep a copy of the protocol you have helped to develop in your portfolio.

---

**Case study 9.2 continued**

The fail-safe mechanism for Mrs Muddle had been her appointment for a cervical smear. Atrophic vaginitis was evident on examination. On your recommendation, the GP prescribed local oestrogen therapy and the symptoms subsided.

At review six months after the changes were made, you find that the practice staff understand better the importance of following up negative investigations. The changes in recording the MSU results and methods of passing on the information to patients are working well. The practice staff feel, and patients and other staff confirm, that they have become more helpful in directing patients appropriately. You and other health professionals are more aware, and more proactive, about best practice in managing patients with urogenital atrophy.

---

# Example cycle of evidence 9.2

- Focus: maintaining good medical practice
- Other relevant foci: working with colleagues, relationships with patients

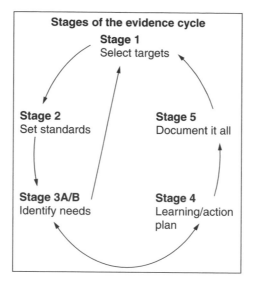

**Stages of the evidence cycle**

**Stage 1**
Select targets

**Stage 2**
Set standards

**Stage 3A/B**
Identify needs

**Stage 4**
Learning/action
plan

**Stage 5**
Document it all

**Case study 9.3**

Mrs Manager is 56 years old. She has been taking a sequential hormone pack for seven years and attends for a routine review. She is happy with her treatment and wishes to continue. However, she has had irregular bleeding and is annoyed when you tell her that this means she will have to return to see the doctor. She explains impatiently to you that she often manipulates the timing of her bleed, as it is more convenient to do that in her busy life. She tells you that she sees no point in having a nurse-led clinic if the nurse has to send patients back to the doctor.

This is just an example. Keep your task simple. You could choose three or four cycles of evidence to demonstrate your competence each year.

## *Stage 1: Select your aspirations for good practice*

The excellent nurse:

- keeps his or her knowledge and skills up to date throughout their working life, through continuing educational activities that maintain and develop competence and performance
- works with colleagues to monitor and maintain the quality of care provided
- takes part in regular and systematic clinical audit and makes improvements accordingly.

## *Stage 2: Set the standards for your outcomes*

Outcomes might include:

- the way learning is applied
- a learnt skill
- a protocol
- a strategy that is implemented
- meeting recommended standards.

- Demonstrate best practice in the management of patients requiring HRT.
- Deliver accurate information to patients.
- Identify the boundaries of your clinical expertise and recognise when to refer on to medical colleagues.

## *Stage 3A: Identify your learning needs*

- Compare your practice with best current practice in the provision of HRT and recommended length of treatment.
- Review the nature and quality of patient education materials including the availability of literature.
- Ask for feedback for medical colleagues on the appropriateness of patients you refer.

## *Stage 3B: Identify your service needs*

Any of the needs assessment exercises in 3A may also reveal service needs.

- Audit the use of sequential HRT in the practice, including setting standards. For example you might agree that 100% of women continuing on HRT should have had a discussion about transferring to continuous combined therapy between the

ages of 52 and 55 years and 100% being reviewed after the age of 52 years should have had a discussion to determine if treatment is still required.
• Discuss with relevant staff the guidelines for the use of HRT.
• Undertake a prospective audit of patients whom you refer back to the GP: follow up these patients through discussion with the GP to see whether you could have managed these cases without referral.

## Stage 4: Make and carry out a learning and action plan

• Perform a literature search for recent recommendations, especially any systematic reviews, for current best practice on HRT.
• Obtain guidelines for running a menopause clinic from an authoritative source, e.g. the British Menopause Society.[27]

## Stage 5: Document your learning, competence, performance and standards of service delivery

• Incorporate and disseminate new information in the guidelines for the menopause clinic.
• Re-audit the use of sequential HRT to confirm that the changes agreed are being implemented.

---

**Case study 9.3 continued**

Mrs Manager visits the GP who tells her that a trial without her HRT treatment is recommended to establish whether she still has symptoms that require treatment and whether she has irregular bleeding when not taking the HRT (as that would require investigation). She is displeased with the change to her routine. The GP asks her to contact you again to discuss the alternatives and for a list of websites and patient information leaflets that will further explain the rationale behind this recommendation.

You and the GP discuss Mrs Manager's future care and decide on a joint policy to maintain a consistent approach. You feel that you will be able to give advice more authoritatively in the future bolstered by your new knowledge and the back-up from other members of the practice team.

---

## Example cycle of evidence 9.3

- Focus: relationship with patients
- Other relevant focus: working with colleagues

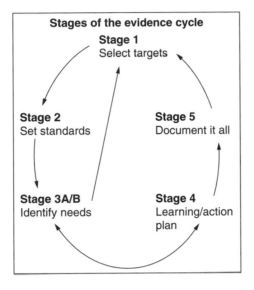

**Stages of the evidence cycle**

**Stage 1**
Select targets

**Stage 2**
Set standards

**Stage 5**
Document it all

**Stage 3A/B**
Identify needs

**Stage 4**
Learning/action plan

---

**Case study 9.3 continued**

Mrs Manager wonders why she was not informed about the availability of patient literature before now. You tell her that patient care is continually improving and adapting to ensure that patients have the opportunity to become experts in their own care. You apologise for not ensuring that she received this information on her previous attendance.

You discuss Mrs Manager with the doctor. Both of you feel that the patient–nurse or patient–doctor interactions with this assertive woman, who is always in a hurry, have affected the quality of care that she has received. You also arrange for the same sources of patient information to be available in the consulting rooms of both doctors and nurses, and ask the healthcare assistant to restock this when supplies become low.

This is just an example. Keep your task simple. You could choose three or four cycles of evidence to demonstrate your competence each year.

## Stage 1: Select your aspirations for good practice

The excellent nurse:

- empowers patients to take informed decisions about their management
- apologises appropriately when things go wrong, and has an adequate complaint procedure in place.

## Stage 2: Set the standards for your outcomes

Outcomes might include:

- the way learning is applied
- a learnt skill
- a protocol
- a strategy that is implemented
- meeting recommended standards.

- Demonstrate consistent best practice in patient relationships.
- Demonstrate that you recognise when your management has not gone as well as it should, apologise appropriately to patient and take steps to remedy the deficiency.

## Stage 3A: Identify your learning needs

- Record in your reflective diary types of nurse–patient interaction that create barriers to best management from feedback from patients.

## Stage 3B: Identify your service needs

Any of the needs assessment exercises in 3A may also reveal service needs.

- Enable colleagues, and staff for whom you are responsible, to recognise and attempt to remove the barriers to best management.
- Undertake a 360° survey within clinicians and practice manager of the practice team, enquiring particularly about colleagues' perceived relationships with patients.
- Review the organisation of nurse-led clinics to identify whether doctors can be available (with some empty appointment slots or while doing administrative duties) to provide advice during clinics.

## Stage 4: Make and carry out a learning and action plan

- Ask a colleague who has done assertiveness training to facilitate role-play scenarios of difficult patient–staff interactions. The scenarios are to include those where the

patient is very authoritative, resulting in the staff member behaving in a subservient or resentful manner.
- Learn how to use that recognition of nurse–patient interaction to modify your consultation style appropriately.
- Use reflective writing with an established reflective model to analyse your interactions with other authoritative patients and record your conclusions about your improvement. [28]

*Stage 5: Document your learning, competence, performance and standards of service delivery*
- Include your reflections and analysis within your portfolio.
- Keep copies of the patient and 360° surveys and subsequent planned changes.

---

**Case study 9.3 continued**

You feel that you have identified and learnt how to improve your management of powerful patients who want rapid consultations and high levels of information.

You develop a much better rapport with Mrs Manager as you review her health needs and recognise that she has learnt to appear busy in order not to be challenged.

---

# Example cycle of evidence 9.4

- Focus: working with colleagues
- Other relevant focus: teaching and training

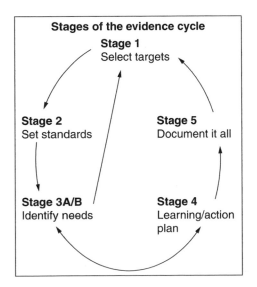

---

**Case study 9.4**

The Primary Care Organisation (PCO) nursing manager asks if you would advise practice nurses on how to set up and run menopause clinics as the PCO is committed to improving and widening the provision of sexual health services.

---

This is just an example. Keep your task simple. You could choose three or four cycles of evidence to demonstrate your competence each year.

## *Stage 1: Select your aspirations for good practice*

The excellent nurse:
- in relationships with colleagues:
  - is supportive to others undertaking a similar role
  - recognises the need to share clinical expertise
  - engages in clinical supervision
- in teaching and training:
  - contributes willingly to the education of students or colleagues
  - develops the skills, attitudes and practices of a competent teacher if he/she has responsibilities for teaching
  - employs the principles of giving accurate feedback to enhance the performance of others.

## *Stage 2: Set the standards for your outcomes*

Outcomes might include:

- the way learning is applied
- a learnt skill
- a protocol
- a strategy that is implemented
- meeting recommended standards.

- Demonstrate and communicate consistent best practice in providing clinical care for menopausal problems.
- Demonstrate and communicate consistent best practice in providing services for patients who require advice and treatment for menopausal problems.

## Stage 3A: Identify your learning needs

- Review the feedback you have received from students on courses, workshops and individual learning sessions that you have run in the last 12 months, and reflect on any learning needs revealed.
- Ask for peer review for the course material you have written for training.
- Check by comparing against guidelines that the knowledge and skills you are imparting are up to date and best practice.

## Stage 3B: Identify your service needs

> Any of the needs assessment exercises in 3A may also reveal service needs.

- Find out what additional help will be available to these nurses and how the PCO intends to help practice nurses develop new clinical skills.
- Discuss how the dual demands of service provision and education needs of new practice nurses can be effectively merged.
- Establish a group of interested health professionals with expertise in the menopause, who can help take this initiative forward rather than attempting to carry the load alone.

## Stage 4: Make and carry out a learning and action plan

- Undertake a refresher teaching and assessing course to ensure an optimal approach to students and junior staff.
- Approach the nursing department within the local university to see if they would consider developing an accredited course for nurses on managing the menopause.
- Write, and obtain feedback on, training materials for the topic.
- Read widely about the subject of the menopause, both literature for nurses and patients.
- Arrange for practice nurses to attend your clinic as observers. This will help you to establish what their learning needs might be.

## Stage 5: Document your learning, competence, performance and standards of service delivery

- Record the feedback from nurses who attend your menopause clinic as observers.
- Log the feedback on your teaching, training and written materials.

---

**Case study 9.4 continued**

You establish an expert advisory group where everyone agrees to contribute to the education of practice nurses who are interested in running menopause clinics. The university is more than happy to develop a course with the help of local clinicians and plans to include a variety of educational processes including seminars and clinical placement opportunities, and use a problem-based learning approach to encourage analysis of case histories.

---

# References

1  Bungay GT, Vessey MP and McPherson CK (1980) Study of symptoms in middle life with special reference to the menopause. *British Medical Journal.* **281**: 181–3.

2  Nugent D and Balen A (1999) Pregnancy in the older woman. *Journal of the British Menopause Society.* **5**: 132–4.

3  Brechin S and Gebbie A (1999) *Perimenopausal Contraception: FACT review.* www.ffprhc.org.uk

4  Hunter MS (1996) Depression and menopause. *British Medical Journal.* **313**: 1217–18.

5  Nicol-Smith L (1996) Causality, menopause, and depression: A critical review of the literature. *British Medical Journal.* **313**: 1229–32.

6  Woods NF and Sullivan EM (1997) Pathways to depressed mood in midlife women: observations from the Seattle Women's Health Study. *Research in Nursing and Health.* **20**: 119–29.

7  Anonymous (1999) *Osteoporosis. Clinical guidelines for prevention and treatment.* Royal College of Physicians, London.

8  Black DM, Steinbuch M, Palermo L *et al.* (2001) An assessment tool for predicting fracture risk in postmenopausal women. *Osteoporosis International.* **12**: 519–28.

9  Guthrie JR (1999) Role of lifestyle approaches in the management of the menopause. *Journal of the British Menopause Society.* **5**: 25–8.

10  Ernst E (1999) Herbal remedies as a treatment of some frequent symptoms during menopause. *Journal of the British Menopause Society.* **5**: 117–20.

11  Davis SR (2001) Phytoestrogen therapy for menopausal symptoms? *British Medical Journal.* **323**: 354–5.

12  www.acupuncture.org.uk/content/Library/menopause_bp5.pdf

13  Bandolier (1998) Alternatives for the menopause. *Bandolier.* **56**: 3 and on www.jr2.ox.ac.uk/bandolier/band56/b56-3.html

14  Rees M, Purdie D and Hope S (2003) *The Menopause. What you need to know.* BMS Publications, Marlow.

15  Committee on Safety of Medicines (September 2003) HRT: update on the risk of breast cancer and long-term safety. *Current Problems in Pharmacovigilance.* **29**: 1–3. www.mca.gov.uk

16  Pitkin J, Rees MCP, Gray S *et al.* (2003) Managing the menopause. British Menopause Society Council Consensus statement on hormone replacement therapy. *Journal of British Menopause Society.* **9(3)**: 129–31.

17   Panay N (2004) Hormone replacement therapy: the way forward. *Journal of Family Planning and Reproductive Health Care.* **30(1)**: 21–3.

18   Rymer J, Wilson R and Ballard K (2003) Making decisions about hormone replacement therapy. *British Medical Journal.* **326**: 322–6.

19   Collaborative Group on Hormonal Factors in Breast Cancer (1997) Breast cancer and hormone replacement therapy: collaborative reanalysis of data from 51 epidemiological studies of 52 705 women with breast cancer and 108 411 women without breast cancer. *Lancet.* **350**: 1047–59.

20   Writing Group for the Women's Health Initiative Investigators (2002) Risks and benefits of estrogen plus progestin in healthy postmenopausal women: principal results from the Women's Health Initiative randomized controlled trial. *Journal of the American Medical Association.* **288**: 321–33.

21   Million Women Study Collaborators (2003) Breast cancer and hormone replacement therapy in the Million Women Study. *Lancet.* **362**: 419–27.

22   Buckler HM, Kalsi PK, Cantrill JA and Anderson DC (1995) An audit of oestradiol levels and implant frequency in women undergoing subcutaneous implant therapy. *Clinical Endocrinology.* **42(5)**: 445–50.

23   Davis SR (2003) Menopause: new therapies. *Menopause Journal of Australia.* **178(12)**: 634–7. Full text available with references on www.mja.com.au

24   Raudaskoski T, Tapanainen J, Tomas E *et al.* (2002) Intrauterine 10 microgram and 20 microgram levonorgestrel systems in postmenopausal women receiving oral oestrogen therapy: clinical endometrial and metabolic response. *British Journal of Obstetrics and Gynaecology.* **109**: 135–44.

25   Rees M and Purdie DW (eds) (2002) *Management of the Menopause* (3e). The British Menopause Society, Marlow.

26   Morris E and Rymer J (2003) Menopausal symptoms. *Clinical Evidence Concise.* **10**: 398–9 and www.clinicalevidence.com

27   www.the-bms.org

28   Schon D (1983) *The Reflective Practitioner: how professionals think in action.* Basic Books, New York.

# Further reading and resources

- Rees M and Purdie DW (eds) (2002) *Management of the Menopause* (3e). BMS Publications Ltd, Marlow. This publication contains a large number of references and suggestions for further reading on all aspects of the menopause.

- www.the-bms.org and the *Journal of the British Menopause Society* give information to help to keep you up to date with new information and controversies.

- www.menopausematters.co.uk offers practical information on the menopause and HRT, including subjects like contraception in the perimenopause. The clinician-led site is aimed mainly at patients, but also has a section aimed at health professionals who want to keep up with their patients!

# 10

## Teenager-friendly healthcare

**Case study 10.1**

Miss Tean is 16 years old. She attends the 'healthy teenager' clinic, which has been set up as a drop-in centre where adolescents can access confidential healthcare advice. She appears rather vague and you are not sure why she has come to see you. She tells you that her mother thought she should have a 'check up'.

## What issues you should cover

Teenagers often find the prospect of visiting a health professional very daunting. Do not underestimate how difficult it may have been for Miss Tean to pluck up courage to come and see you. Show an interest in her health. What might appear as minor issues to you might be a major cause of concern to her. Nurses are generally perceived as less threatening than doctors, but as this may be the first time that she has consulted a health professional without a parent being present to speak for her it may be a major step in the journey to adulthood. If you are able to remove some of her embarrassment with an open relaxed approach this could positively influence her attitude to all health professionals. Adolescence is known to be a time of low confidence and awkwardness in new situations is common. Try to address this by giving plenty of information and giving clear direction about what you need to know to establish a baseline health profile.

Always start by introducing yourself – using your first name will lower any perceived imbalance of power and put the two of you on a more equal footing. Briefly explaining your role will also be helpful to help her understand the set-up of the clinic, e.g. 'I'm a nurse with a special interest in teenagers' problems, but although I can give you lots of advice I can't actually prescribe any treatment, but I can ask the doctor to do that if we feel it's necessary'. You may need to positively build up her trust in you if she is fearful about any lack of privacy or confidentiality in the practice. Your good relationship may help to reinforce your healthcare advice and encourage her compliance with any treatments you recommend.

## Structure the consultation

If Miss Tean is not admitting to any obvious reason for the consultation, you can take this opportunity to undertake a health screen that will allow for preventive health-care advice. Explain what this will involve, i.e. that you will check weight and height, record blood pressure, undertake a routine urine test and check out how healthy her current lifestyle is. After outlining what you intend to do, check that this is acceptable with Miss Tean and ask if there is anything else that she would like you to cover. Several invitations to discuss anything else may reassure her that it is OK to ask about something that is on her mind.

Whilst undertaking the screening procedures, remember to tell Miss Tean why you are doing them, e.g. by measuring both your height and weight we can match these up together to see if you fit in the category of 'very healthy' or whether there is something we could do to improve your health. This approach emphasises the partnership in healthcare and you are teaching the patient what to expect in future healthcare provision. Emphasising when results are normal is reassuring to everyone – but may be particularly helpful with adolescents who frequently think they are different from everyone else! Encourage Miss Tean to fully participate in the consultation by asking 'open' questions. It is easy to forget to do this when you have determined on a set agenda of screening. However, rather than the traditional approach of 'Do you smoke? Do you drink' etc, try a more open approach such as 'Tell me about your smoking and drinking habits' or 'Tell me about anything you do that you think might be unhealthy'.

## Talking about sex

Raising the issue of sex with teenagers can feel awkward at first. Develop some techniques to help you feel confident with this. It will certainly be something they have thought about! If you don't broach the subject they may not have the courage to do so – and a golden opportunity for advice could be lost.

Asking about periods is a good introduction because it moves towards a more personal side of healthcare. It is rare for teenagers to always have completely regular periods, but they do not always appreciate this. A short discussion about hormonal changes during the menstrual cycle may help them to understand that this is a complex process and is subject to many fluctuations within the first few years of menarche. However, do not allow them to think that they do not need to worry if they miss a period if they have had unprotected sex!

Taking a full sexual history is probably not appropriate or necessary during a routine 'screening' consultation such as this.[1] However, establishing whether the patient is sexually active is important, as this will also require questions and information-giving around contraception to ensure they are adequately protected against unwanted pregnancy (*see* Chapter 5). Raising teenagers' awareness of risk factors associated with sexual behaviour is also important. Rates of STIs as a consequence of not using barrier methods of contraception are soaring in young people.[2] Although it is important to adopt a non-judgemental attitude, it is also important not to condone behaviour that will put teenagers at risk. It may be appropriate to check that they feel 'in control' of their sexual relationships, emphasising that the need to feel good about what you are doing is a major component of sexual satisfaction.

Teenagers should all have experienced some type of sex education at school although parents are at liberty to withdraw children from sex education when this is not part of the national curriculum.[3] The Education Act of 1996 stipulates that education on hormonal contraception and STIs must be included as part of the science curriculum.[4] This means that parents cannot withdraw their children from these elements of sex education, as science is a core subject.

Many schools will be delighted to engage the assistance of nurses in developing or delivering teaching on sex education. Many school nurses are actively involved in sex and relationship education with schools and this has real advantages in crossing the health–education divide. However, nurses who do become involved with this subject in schools will need to be fully familiar with the Fraser guidelines (*see* Chapter 3) and ensure that confidentiality is upheld at all times.[5] This is most easily done by explaining your position as a health professional and emphasising that it would be inappropriate to comment on individual problems in a classroom situation.

## Encouraging young people to adopt a healthy lifestyle

Advice on healthy lifestyles will not differ dramatically from the advice given for any age group (*see* Chapter 4), although the manner in which issues are tackled is likely to differ. Examples of how to live a healthy life will need to alter in line with the age group. Warn against the dangers of anorexia nervosa and emphasise the normal range of BMI for those who appear overly concerned about weight which falls within normal parameters. Remember that teenagers do not often do the cooking at home so advice on low fat foods, etc, should be included in literature that they can take home for their parents to read. However, they may appreciate being informed about the relative fat content of frequently consumed fast foods or snacks.

If you discover that Miss Tean smokes cigarettes and that she is also on the contraceptive pill, remember to review her safety and discuss her risks with her. Oral contraceptives have been shown to have an adverse effect on deaths from ischaemic heart disease only in women who were currently smoking 15 or more cigarettes per day.[6]

Miss Tean has presented to you with a vague remit of 'wanting a check up', and although this may be a genuine reason for consultation it is also important to recognise that there may be underlying problems that she finds difficult to raise. A study of 700 young people in the West Midlands explored the range of clinical conditions that usually bring young people to see their GP.[7,8] The reasons for consultations with GPs are listed in Table 10.1. Teenagers may well consult with a dermatological condition such as acne, but have an underlying mental health problem that they conceal or of which they are unaware. It is startling how few young people consulted their GPs with a psychological condition or other mental health problem in this study and it is likely that this finding applies elsewhere in the UK.

Teenagers like Miss Tean tend to present lots of health queries if encouraged by the interest of their GP or practice nurse. Table 10.2 describes how frequently young people consulted health professionals and others for common conditions.[8] Teenagers

**Table 10.1:**   Reasons for consultation with a GP, over a 12-month period (total number = 700 young people)[7]

| Condition | Number per hundred |
|---|---|
| Respiratory | 35 |
| Dermatological | 28 |
| Musculoskeletal | 22 |
| Otorhinological | 18 |
| Urogenital | 9 |
| Gastrointestinal | 8 |
| Psychological | 4 |
| Ophthalmic | 4 |
| Miscellaneous | 14 |

**Table 10.2:**   Types of people consulted for different health conditions by 15–16 year olds[8]

| Condition | Percentages of professionals or others consulted for specific conditions | | | | |
|---|---|---|---|---|---|
| | No one | GP | School nurse | Clinic staff | Other |
| Spots/acne | 39 | 51 | 1 | 5 | 4 |
| Diet | 50 | 31 | 9 | 4 | 7 |
| Smoking | 64 | 16 | 9 | 3 | 8 |
| Pregnancy | 34 | 25 | 4 | 30 | 5 |
| STIs | 58 | 18 | 9 | 8 | 6 |

were most likely to go to their GP for skin complaints and least likely to go to the GP in respect of smoking or STIs. The very high numbers of young people not using any source of advice from a health professional is a serious cause of concern.[7,8]

In this study, the GP seemed to be over-used in comparison with other health professionals in areas where they could offer an equivalent level of knowledge and care (e.g. diet, smoking, STIs). It may be necessary for nurses to more actively promote their skills with teenagers in primary care settings, as this may encourage a more collaborative approach to healthcare. One study of general practices in Nottingham showed that increased nurse time was associated with a lower teenage pregnancy rate.[9] Another research study showed that few teenagers received health promotion advice or information from their general practice teams, so the practices involved set up new opportunities for consultations with practice nurses. Teenagers who attended welcomed the consultations with practice nurses to discuss health concerns and develop plans for healthier lifestyles. The consultations provided an effective opportunity to identify and tackle mental and physical health problems and encourage healthy lifestyles. Change in behaviour was slight but encouraging, and the intervention was well received and relatively cheap.[10]

Another important feature of a healthy lifestyle is limiting alcohol. Although Miss Tean is only 16 years old, she is likely to be drinking alcohol. Statistics tell us that just over half (53%) of 15–16-year-old girls and 58% of boys of the same age will have had so much alcohol as to be 'really drunk' on at least two occasions; 15% of girls and 21% of boys will have done so on more than 10 occasions.[11,12] Other surveys have corroborated these findings. Drinking alcohol at parties and friends' houses is a normal part of the social life of a teenager. Drinking alcohol increases the likelihood of having sex, and reduces the likelihood of using contraception. One survey of 16–19 year olds found that 19% reported that, after drinking alcohol, they had had sex that they had later regretted, and 10% said they had had unsafe sex after drinking alcohol.[13]

## Providing teenager-friendly services

You need to look at all aspects of the way services are provided for Miss Tean and her peers. Look at the information they have when they are considering making an appointment, what flexibility exists in booking a consultation, especially in an emergency, and how welcoming is the atmosphere of the waiting room and staff? Consider the way in which the healthcare team involves teenagers in making decisions about options for treatment, and the resources used for sharing information about health matters. Look at staff communication skills with young people and how arrangements for follow up are made. The attitudes of receptionists are particularly important for this group who may be easily be put off by an overly inquisitive or officious attitude.

A study of communication with teenagers in general practice found that they wanted: [14]

- flexible, non-embarrassing access to non-judgemental healthcare
- time to explore reasons for attending within the primary care consultation
- information not lectures
- explanations in plain English and not medical jargon
- to be treated with the same respect as adults
- to be made aware of their choices in healthcare
- to be made aware of the duties of health professionals and the rights of patients e.g. confidentiality.

The study revealed a conflict between what GPs and teenagers viewed as being 'good' communication. GPs judged good communication as being the teenager listening to the GP, taking advice, being passive and not causing trouble. Teenagers thought good communication was being given time to explain their problems in their own way, having their health problems explained to them in language they understand and being made to feel legitimate patients. Young people studied did not believe promises of confidentiality made by health professionals, citing their collective experiences of breaches in confidentiality.[14] This study has important implications for nurses who have an opportunity to learn to improve on the reported deficiencies in communication skills of their medical colleagues!

## Tips for providing services to teenagers[15,16]

- Discuss the practice guidelines on confidentiality with all young people (*see* Chapter 3) and make it a priority issue in the practice.

- Always offer the young person the option of being seen alone.
- Follow up young people more frequently initially to build up their trust and confidence and answer their questions and concerns.
- Know the local policies and procedures for child protection, in case you find out that a young person is at risk of suffering or significant harm.
- Know and follow the Fraser recommendations for advice and prescription for the under-16 year olds (*see* Chapter 3).[5]
- Involve school nurses as part of the integrated provision of health advice and contraceptive services in your district.
- Provide an easily accessible help service that young people can contact for advice that they trust. This might be provided by nurses working within a general practice setting or by school nurses, and could involve drop-in clinics, or alternatives to face-to-face consultations. You could advertise an electronic resource to offer answers to common queries about sex and other health issues. Links could be provided from school or practice websites to other useful information, e.g. for the Connexions website[17] or the 'teenage health freak' website.[18]
- Encourage practice teams to look at ways to promote a teenager-friendly environment. Ask teenagers themselves for their views about what works.
- Identify the characteristics of the 10–18 year olds in your area of practice so you can plan to address their needs – boys as well as girls.
- Improve the knowledge base of nurses and receptionists about contraception as appropriate – all have their role to play in their interaction with teenagers coming in for contraception.
- Inform young people about what is provided in local practices by posters, a practice information booklet for teenagers, and 'birthday' letters to all young people on practice lists when they become 16 years old (or earlier).
- Advertise services that are available for young people outside of the immediate area.
- Consider organising a young person's clinic run at convenient times for teenagers.
- Involve parents in provision of services for young people and in compiling information for parents about teenagers' health.
- Offer advice and support for teenagers who do get pregnant, providing information about, and referral to, supporting agencies.

# How you can make an impact on young people's risk-taking behaviour

Concentrate on controlling the most common sources of risk in primary care. These include poor continuity of care, communication difficulties and informing virgins about emergency contraception. Work with teachers and parents to give them accurate information about contraception that they in turn can relay to young people. Provide information to debunk common myths that tempt young people to take unnecessary risks.

Focus on health promotion messages about safe sex whenever a young person comes for emergency contraception – safe from pregnancy, safe from infection and safe from coercion. Establish a good rapport in the emergency situation and the young person will return for more routine care when you can discuss health risks associated with smoking, excessive alcohol and substance misuse too. Tell young people more about the subsequent effects of sexual infection such as the increased rates of infertility from infection with *Chlamydia* and the association of alcohol and drug misuse with unwanted pregnancy. Learn more about how to motivate teenagers to resist or reduce risky behaviour.

Make sure that your health promotion literature is reproduced in all the languages of your patient population. For instance, the manufacturers of the progesterone depot injection produce patient information leaflets in English, Greek, Bengali, Hindi, Chinese, Punjabi, Urdu, Gujarati and Turkish.

# Collecting data to demonstrate your learning, competence, performance and standards of service delivery

## Example cycle of evidence 10.1

- Focus: working with colleagues
- Other relevant foci: relationships with patients, teaching and training

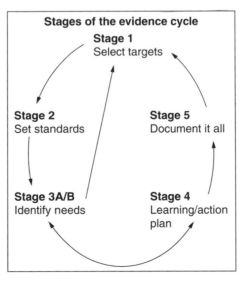

**Stages of the evidence cycle**

Stage 1
Select targets

Stage 2
Set standards

Stage 5
Document it all

Stage 3A/B
Identify needs

Stage 4
Learning/action plan

---

**Case study 10.2**

You are the education lead in your practice team and share responsibility for organising quarterly in-house learning events. The team suggested that you focus on healthcare for teenagers at the next practice team workshop.

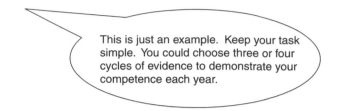

*This is just an example. Keep your task simple. You could choose three or four cycles of evidence to demonstrate your competence each year.*

## Stage 1: Select your aspirations for good practice

The excellent nurse:

- understands the health needs of the local teenage population and tries to ensure that the primary care team has skills to meet those needs.

## Stage 2: Set the standards for your outcomes

Outcomes might include:

- the way learning is applied
- a learnt skill
- a protocol
- a strategy that is implemented
- meeting recommended standards.

- A profile of the health needs of the teenagers registered with the practice.
- An assessment of the learning needs of all members of the primary care team about the provision of healthcare for teenagers.

## Stage 3A: Identify your learning needs

- Find out the statistics about mental and physical morbidity, teenage pregnancy or STIs from national and local public health sources and compare it with what is known from your local practice data.
- Review the records of 20 or more teenagers opportunistically or from a systematic sample. Compare the reasons for consultation with those given in the West Midlands survey in Table 10.1. You could also compare the treatment provided to the teenagers in your survey against best practice.
- Consider if you know how to carry out a learning needs assessment of others in the practice team. Obtain their views afterwards about your approach.

## Stage 3B: Identify your service needs

> Any of the needs assessment exercises in 3A may also reveal service needs.

- Arrange for all relevant members of the practice team to self-assess their learning and training needs. Encourage them to compare this with their job descriptions and with the skills needed for the services you provide or aim to provide in the near future.
- Undertake an audit using a semi-structured short questionnaire to ask clinicians from local pharmacies or family planning clinics, or youth workers at youth clubs about their perceptions of local services. Include questions about the choice of staff, availability and accessibility of female or male doctors or nurses, the timing and convenience of services, and whether they receive comments about the atmosphere at various healthcare premises.

## Stage 4: Make and carry out a learning and action plan

- Update, or write, clinical protocols for teenagers who have asthma or diabetes. Look up best practice in management, patient choice, and the legal aspects of consent and confidentiality. This might include reading and reflection, searching the literature or reading a review in a peer reviewed journal, downloading a recommended protocol by a nationally recognised organisation, or a discussion with peers at a topic-based group.
- Obtain public health data about the morbidity of the teenage population and discuss it with colleagues at staff meetings or in a special interest group of the PCO.
- Plan the in-house learning event around the information you have gathered in Stage 3 and the updated clinical protocols that have been customised for the special needs of teenagers.

## Stage 5: Document your learning, competence, performance and standards of service delivery.

- Audit the adherence to the updated practice protocols.
- Include the programme for the in-house learning event and the subsequent action plan in your portfolio.
- Distribute the health profile of the teenage practice population with information from as many sources as possible for discussion at future staff events.

---

**Case study 10.2 continued**

After your in-house training event, a few people volunteer to find out more from teenagers about their needs and preferences in the way you provide healthcare. You agree to start with teenagers who have asthma or diabetes.

# Example cycle of evidence 10.2

- Focus: teaching and training
- Other relevant focus: confidentiality

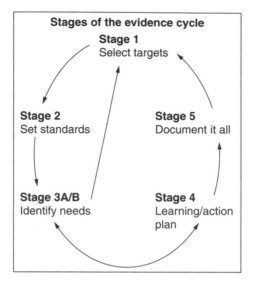

**Stages of the evidence cycle**

Stage 1
Select targets

Stage 2
Set standards

Stage 5
Document it all

Stage 3A/B
Identify needs

Stage 4
Learning/action plan

---

**Case study 10.3**

Laura Fear asks whether details of her consultation really are confidential in view of the fact that her father is a GP in a local practice. She said she has been unsure about coming to see you, and wondered whether she should attend a family planning clinic in the city centre as, despite this being a bus-ride away, she knows they welcome 15 year olds like herself.

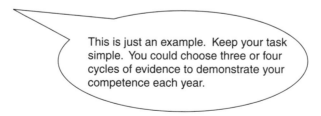

This is just an example. Keep your task simple. You could choose three or four cycles of evidence to demonstrate your competence each year.

*Stage 1: Select your aspirations for good practice*

The excellent nurse:

- has a personal commitment to teaching and learning
- keeps patients' information confidential – including maintaining privacy to make sure that confidential information is not overheard.

*Stage 2: Set the standards for your outcomes*

---

Outcomes might include:

- the way learning is applied
- a learnt skill
- a protocol
- a strategy that is implemented
- meeting recommended standards.

---

- Ensure that all members of the practice team, including you, new members of staff, and students, are familiar with guidelines for confidentiality in relation to young people receiving healthcare.

*Stage 3A: Identify your learning needs*

- Self-assess your knowledge, and check that of team members, about the guidelines for confidentiality for providing under-16 year olds with contraception or referring for termination of pregnancy.
- Request a staff training session on maintaining confidentiality for teenagers of different ages, and offer to be involved in the organisation of this. Suggest a workshop approach so that everyone can feel involved as this will be more likely to lead to change where necessary.

*Stage 3B: Identify your service needs*

---

Any of the needs assessment exercises in 3A may also reveal service needs.

---

- Compare your protocol for confidentiality with the guidelines in the *Confidentiality and Young People* toolkit.[19]
- Review the induction programme for new members of staff (including administrative staff), students on placement, and doctors in training to assess the extent to which knowledge of confidentiality features.

*Stage 4: Make and carry out a learning and action plan*

- Find out how to establish the learning needs in an interactive multidisciplinary group from books or from a tutor.[20,21]
- Prepare for and run an interactive session on confidentiality with a special focus on teenagers. Invite others in the practice team, students, family planning or school nurses, local pharmacists, specialist nurses, GPs etc. You might use the *Confidentiality and Young People* toolkit to stimulate discussion.[19]

*Stage 5: Document your learning, competence, performance and standards of service delivery*

- Keep a copy of the summary of the results of a quiz completed by those attending the interactive session, comparing their answers before and afterwards.
- Include records of any reported or perceived breaches of confidentiality by anyone working in the practice (suitably anonymised) and how this could be avoided in future.
- Keep a copy of the personal learning plans for new staff by the end of the induction period.

---

**Case study 10.3 continued**

Miss Fear is reassured when you explain about the nurses' professional code of conduct and the need to maintain confidentiality. Explain that this is maintained unless this puts her or anyone else at significant risk. Then medical information may need to be shared with others after seeking her consent. You tell her that you would expect none of the staff to mention that she has been to see you at all – now or in the future. You check that everyone has attended the in-house training on confidentiality and then advertise this fact within the waiting room.

---

# Example cycle of evidence 10.3

- Focus: management
- Other relevance focus: relationships with colleagues

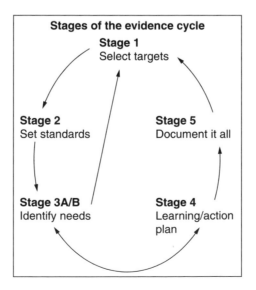

**Stages of the evidence cycle**

**Stage 1**
Select targets

**Stage 2**
Set standards

**Stage 5**
Document it all

**Stage 3A/B**
Identify needs

**Stage 4**
Learning/action plan

> **Case study 10.4**
> You are the lead health professional in your practice team for sexual health. Your PCO has called upon you to represent your practice and work with other practice leads to re-configure contraceptive services in your practice so that they are appropriate for the needs of young people.

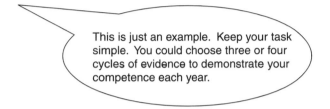

This is just an example. Keep your task simple. You could choose three or four cycles of evidence to demonstrate your competence each year.

## *Stage 1: Select your aspirations for good practice*

The excellent nurse:

* strives to address the health priorities of the patient population in collaboration with the PCO – in relation to teenage contraception.

## *Stage 2: Select the standards for your outcomes*

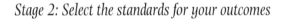

Outcomes might include:

* the way learning is applied
* a learnt skill
* a protocol
* a strategy that is implemented
* meeting recommended standards.

* Re-configure the contraceptive services in the practice to provide them in ways appropriate for the needs and preferences of young people.

## *Stage 3A: Identify your learning needs*

* Self-assess your knowledge of which characteristics of young people put them most at risk of unplanned teenage pregnancy. Include assessment of knowledge about trends in sexual activity and the use of contraceptives during the teen years.
* Get recent statistics of the conception rates for your practice area from the local public health lead. Compare them with practice data about live births and termination rates.

*Stage 3B: Identify your service needs*

> Any of the needs assessment exercises in 3A may also reveal service needs.

- Run a search to find out how prescribing rates of contraceptives differ for teenagers living in various geographical areas.
- Compare your practice organisation with examples of good practice for making the practice teenager friendly.
- Organise, design and give out a short quiz to all young people coming to the reception desk about what would make them feel welcome and respected in health-care settings and your practice in particular.
- Conduct a significant event audit around three consecutive cases of young people presenting as pregnant. Look at the duration of the pregnancy before consulting for the first time, the age of the teenager, whether the pregnancy was planned, whether contraception had been used previously and the reasons for the failure or non-use of contraception.

*Stage 4: Make and carry out a learning and action plan*

- Attend a workshop run by a teenage pregnancy lead to learn about local initiatives and meet others from local authority agencies concerned with teenage health problems.
- Read a book about the provision of contraception to teenagers and reflect on the changes needed to your current management.[2]
- Represent the practice at a workshop with the public health lead for the PCO and other practice representatives. Help to formulate changes to the way contraceptive services are provided for young people in the local area to meet local needs and preferences.

*Stage 5: Document your learning, competence, performance and standards of service delivery*

- Include a copy of the statistics for conception rates of teenagers in your own practice and across the PCO.
- Report on the changes to contraceptive service provision in the practice and changes in numbers of patients seen.
- Keep a copy of the feedback from teenagers obtaining contraception. This could be obtained by asking them to complete feedback questions slips or from notes of their responses to standard enquiries made by the GP or nurse.

> **Case study 10.4 continued**
>
> Armed with all the information you have gathered, you are able to make a good case for the changes you feel are required in the provision of sexual health services for young people.

# References

1   Sutherland C (2001) Young people and sex. In: G Andrews *Women's Sexual Health* (2e). Baillière Tindall, London.

2   Wakley G and Chambers R (2002) *Sexual Health Matters in Primary Care.* Radcliffe Medical Press, Oxford.

3   Department for Education (1994) *Education Act 1993: sex education in schools.* Circular number 5/94. Department for Education, London.

4   Sex Education Forum (1997) *Ensuring Entitlement: a sex education charter.* Forum factsheet no. 14. National Children's Bureau, London.

5   The Fraser Guidelines (1985) House of Lords Judgement, London.

6   Vessey M, Painter R and Yeates D (2003) Mortality in relation to oral contraceptive use and cigarette smoking. *Lancet.* **362**: 185–91.

7   Jacobson L, Mellanby AR, Donovan C *et al.* (2000) Teenagers' views on general practice consultations and other medical advice. *Family Practice.* **17**: 156–8.

8   Coleman J and Schofield J (2003) *Key Data on Adolescents.* Trust for the Study of Adolescence, TSA Publishing Ltd, Brighton.

9   Hippisley-Cox J, Allen J, Pringle M *et al.* (2000) Association between teenage pregnancy rates and the age and sex of general practitioners: cross sectional survey in Trent 1994–7. *British Medical Journal.* **320**: 842–5.

10  Walker Z, Townsend J, Oakley L *et al.* (2002) Health promotion for adolescents in primary care: randomised controlled trial. *British Medical Journal.* **325**: 524.

11  Churchill R, Allen J, Denman S *et al.* (2000) Do the attitudes and beliefs of young teenagers towards general practice influence actual consultation behaviour? *British Journal of General Practice.* **50**: 953–7.

12  Hasden L, Angle H and Hickman M (1999) *Young People and Health: health behaviour in school-aged children.* A report of 1997 findings. Health Education Authority, London.

13  Eborall C and Garmeson K (2000) *Research to Inform the National Media Campaign.* Teenage Pregnancy Unit, Department of Health, London.

14  MORI (1999) Risk taking among young people. Presentation of qualitative research to Department of Health. Cited in: C Eborall and K Garmeson (2000) *Research to Inform the National Media Campaign.* Teenage Pregnancy Unit, Department of Health, London.

15  Donovan C, Richardson G, Parry-Langdon N and Jacobson L (2001) *Bridging the Gap.* Bro Taf Health Authority, South Wales.

16  MacPherson A, Donovan C and Macfarlane A (2002) *Healthcare of Young People. Promotion in primary care.* Radcliffe Medical Press, Oxford.

17  www.connexions.gov.uk

18   www.teenagehealthfreak.org

19   Donovan C (ed.) (2000) *Confidentiality and Young People. A toolkit for general practice, primary care groups and trusts.* Royal College of General Practitioners and Brook, London.

20   Chambers R, Wakley G, Iqbal Z and Field S (2002) *Prescription for Learning.* Radcliffe Medical Press, Oxford.

21   Mohanna K, Wall D and Chambers R (2003) *Teaching Made Easy* (2e). Radcliffe Medical Press, Oxford.

# And finally

We hope that you have found that the stages in our 'cycle of evidence' are a useful approach to gathering information about what you need to learn. You can also use it to identify improvements you or others need to make to the way you deliver services.

It is easy to feel overwhelmed by having to demonstrate that you are competent and perform consistently well as a nurse in order to re-register with the NMC every three years. Try to get into the habit of reflective writing to learn from critical incidents and include these in your portfolio. Recognise when you have achieved change in practice, and remember to put the documentary evidence in your portfolio. Use the portfolio as a teaching aid with students and junior staff to show that the process of lifelong learning is a reality.

Ask your manager to use your individual performance review to focus you on tasks you could achieve in order to improve practice. Both colleagues and patients will be well placed to help you to set your aspirations for good practice and set achievable standards for your outcomes – of learning and improvements in service delivery. Perhaps your manager can help you to develop learning and action in your PDP. These cycles of evidence will be the nucleus of your PDP. Colleagues can support you in documenting the evidence of your competence, performance and subsequent standards of service delivery. Other books in this series might help you to look at specific clinical areas, especially those where quality frameworks or special interests require your attention. Remember to visit the supporting website for this book, which includes useful website links: www.health.mattersonline.com.

So the evidence will be there ready to submit for appraisal interviews, re-registration, or when applying for a new job, but the results will show what a good nurse you really are. The patients you care for will be the ones to benefit most from your efforts to provide optimal quality. This should give you increasing confidence and self-respect. Enjoy your professional glow.

# Index

360° feedback 17–19, 135, 180–1

abuse, sexual 47, 83
access to healthcare 20, 26, 29, 31, 39
'accredited for prior experiential learning'
    (APEL) 8
Acheson report 83
acne 88, 151, 170, 189–90
action plans 10, 11, 23
acupuncture 56, 166
Addison's disease 151
adverse events 21, 28, 114, 116 *see also*
    significant event audit
Advertising Standards Agency 93
advocacy, nurses' 44, 97, 132, 141
age
    contraception 47, 82
    infertility 122–3
    menopause 163
    population health needs 30
    vaginal bleeding problems 146, 148
Age of Legal Capacity (Scotland) Act 1991
    47
Agenda for Change 15, 24
alcohol
    infertility 123
    menopause 165, 166
    obesity 64
    teenagers 83, 188, 190–1, 193
    women's lifestyle 55, 62–3, 73–6
alopecia 151
Alzheimer's disease 168
amenorrhoea 137–8, 148–52, 172
anaemia 142
androgens 151, 156, 169
angina pectoris 58
anorexia 61, 148–51, 189
antenatal care 66–7, 83
anxiety 56, 61, 163, 166
APEL ('accredited for prior experiential
    learning') 8
appraisal 2–5, 8, 11–12, 16, 203
arthritis 58, 165
assessment 11, 22, 29–32, 36

asthma 12, 195
audiotapes 11, 24, 42, 67, 78, 87
audit
    complaints 52–3
    consent 36, 41–3, 46
    contraception 87
    evidence cycles 68–73, 129
    learning and service needs 20–2, 24,
        26, 29
    PDPs and appraisal 3, 10
    significant event audit 21–2
    STIs 109, 114, 118
azoospermia 126, 131

bacterial vaginosis (BV) 104, 106, 107
bad news, breaking 135–6
best practice
    appraisal vi, 4, 5
    consent 36, 39, 42, 46
    contraception 93, 97
    infertility 129, 132, 135
    learning and service needs 1, 16, 21
    menopause 174, 177–8, 180, 182–3
    STIs 111, 114, 117
    teenagers 194–5
    vaginal bleeding problems 154,
        159–60
    women's lifestyle 67, 72
beta-blockers 125, 126
binge eating 57
birth weight 55, 65–6, 83
bleeding *see* vaginal bleeding problems
blood pressure
    contraception 83, 92, 96
    HRT 168
    women's lifestyle 57–9, 61, 74, 78
blood tests 63, 76, 107–8, 121, 151,
    165–6
body mass index (BMI)
    HRT 168
    infertility 121
    teenagers 189
    vaginal bleeding problems 149–50
    women's lifestyle 57, 58, 60, 72

bone density
    contraception 88
    menopause 165, 167, 169–72
    vaginal bleeding problems 145, 150
    women's lifestyle 77
breakthrough bleeding (BTB) 172
breast cancer 58, 167–9, 171–2
breast examinations 53, 77, 149, 150, 168
breast milk 88, 90, 96, 137, 148, 150
British Menopause Society 172, 178, 185
*British National Formulary* (BNF) 126
Brook Centres 84
buddies 18, 24
BV *see* bacterial vaginosis

CAGE (Cut, Annoyed, Guilty, Eye-opener) questionnaire 63, 74, 76
calcium 150, 165, 168, 171
Caldicott Committee Report 47
cancer
    breast 58, 167–9, 171–2
    cervical 45, 63, 105, 156, 158
    colorectal 58, 168
    endometrium 142, 167, 171, 172
    lungs 55, 56
    ovaries 58, 127, 172
    testicles 126
candida (thrush) 104, 106, 107
carbohydrate, in diet 59
carers 36, 44, 45
cervical cancer 45, 63, 105, 156, 158
cervical ectopy (erosion/ectropion) 152–3, 156–8
cervical smears
    complaints 52–3
    consent 44–6
    infertility 123, 137
    menopause 168, 170, 173, 175
    STIs 105–6, 108
    vaginal bleeding 141, 142, 153, 156–8
    women's health 63–4, 77
child protection 36, 192
*Chlamydia*
    emergency contraception 87
    evidence cycles 116–19
    infertility 124, 126
    pregnancy 115
    screening tests 107–9
    statistics 103–4

teenagers 193
    vaginal bleeding problems 152, 153
cholesterol 59, 61
cirrhosis 105
clinical care (evidence cycles)
    contraception 91–8
    infertility 128–31
    menopause 173–5
    smoking cessation 65–7
    STIs 110–12
    vaginal bleeding problems 153–6
clinical governance 18, 42, 93
clomiphene 127, 131, 133
COC pill *see* combined oral contraceptive pill
*Code of Professional Conduct* (NMC) 1, 4–5, 35, 198
colleagues (working with)
    evidence cycles
        complaints 51–4
        consent 43–6
        contraception 91–8
        infertility 136–8
        menopause 173–84
        miscarriage 159–61
        STIs 113–16
        teenagers 193–5, 198–201
    learning and service needs 16, 17, 23–5, 203
    PDPs and appraisal 11, 12
combined hormone replacement therapy 167, 169–70, 172, 177
combined oral contraceptive (COC) pill 85, 143, 145, 152
communication skills
    complaints 51
    consent 39
    evidence cycles 43–6, 75, 78, 115
    learning and service needs 23, 24, 31
    teenagers 191
competence
    complaints 53
    consent and confidentiality 45, 46
    learning and service needs 15–16, 18, 25, 31
    PDPs and appraisal 4–7, 12
complaints 6, 23, 39–40, 51–4, 97, 180
compliance 37, 169, 187
computers 26, 29, 36, 46, 48, 53, 72
concordance 37
condoms 81–2, 84–5, 103, 123–4, 188

confidentiality
and consent 35–6, 46–50
contraception 81, 196–8
infertility 128–30
learning and service needs 24, 31
PDPs and appraisal 5, 8
STIs 101, 102, 114, 118
teenagers 187, 189, 191, 195–8
*Confidentiality and Young People* toolkit 50,
197
consent
confidentiality 46–8
contraception 38–40, 47, 87
evidence cycles 37–46
in healthcare 35–7
learning disabilities 44–6
learning needs 19, 24
standards 5, 153
STIs 101, 106, 108
teenagers 195, 198
consultations 24, 84, 189–91, 194, 196
continuing professional development (CPD)
1, 3, 8
continuity of care 31, 192
continuous combined HRT 167, 169–70,
172, 177
contraception
condoms 81–2, 84–5, 103, 123–4, 188
confidentiality 46–7, 49, 81, 82
consent 38–40, 47
emergency contraception 38, 40, 81,
85–7, 89, 91–5
implants 39, 87, 88, 97
infertility 122–4
injections 39, 87, 88, 98
IUDs 38–40, 86–9, 96–7, 143, 147
IUS 89, 97–8, 141, 144, 170
menopause 163, 170
oral contraception (pill) 29, 81–3, 85,
90, 93, 98
patches 90
smoking 65–6
sterilisation 89–90, 96–8
teenagers 81–4, 188–9, 191–2,
196–201
vaginal bleeding problems 141, 143,
150, 152–3, 156, 158
vasectomy 89, 90, 97
copper IUDs 87–9, 143
coronary heart disease *see* heart disease

costs evaluation 32–3, 97, 109, 115
counselling
contraception 86, 97–8
infertility 135
miscarriage 160
STIs 109, 114
women's lifestyle 56, 60, 62
CPD *see* continuing professional
development
crime 30, 47, 83
Crohn's disease 165
Cushing's syndrome 151
cycles of evidence *see* evidence cycles
cystic fibrosis 125–6

data protection 36, 48
dementia 45, 168
Department of Health
consent and confidentiality 37, 47
learning and service needs 12, 15
prescribing v, 87
research 42–3
STIs 119
Depo-Provera 87, 88
depression 56, 61, 83, 163, 164, 166
diabetes 12, 57–61, 151–2, 155, 195
diet
bone density 88
infertility 121, 128–9, 131
menopause 165, 166
obesity 55, 57, 59–61, 72, 155
teenagers 83, 189, 190
vaginal bleeding problems 150, 155–6
'well woman' checks 79
disabilities 30, 44–6
discharge 103–6, 137, 152, 156, 158
doctors *see* GPs
drug misuse 30, 46, 75, 83, 193
dysmenorrhoea 89, 141, 144–5
dyspareunia 106, 142, 169, 170
dyspepsia 62, 74, 76
dysuria 104, 105, 106, 173

*E. coli* 103
economic evaluation 32–3
ectopic pregnancy 104, 108, 147–8
ectropion (ectopy/erosion) 152–3, 156–8
Education Act (1996) 189
effectiveness/efficiency 20, 29, 31–3
EIA *see* enzyme immuno-assay tests

emergency contraception
    methods 38, 40, 85–7, 89
    teenagers 81, 91–7, 192
ENB (English National Board) 4
endometrium
    cancer 142, 167, 171, 172
    endometriosis 122, 144–5
    endometritis 106
    menopause 164, 167, 169, 170
    vaginal bleeding problems 144, 153
England, health policies 21, 47, 63, 87
English National Board (ENB) 4
enzyme immuno-assay (EIA) tests 107,
    108, 113
epididymis 90, 104, 126
erosion (ectopy/ectropion) 152–3, 156–8
ethical approval, research 36, 42–3, 117–18
evaluation 28–9, 32–3
evidence cycles *see also* clinical care;
        colleagues; good medical practice;
        patients; teaching and training
    alcohol 73–6
    complaints 51–4
    confidentiality 48–50, 196–8
    consent 37–46
    contraception 91–8, 196–201
    health promotion 76–9
    infertility 128–38
    management 116–19, 198–201
    menopause 173–84
    obesity 70–3
    probity 68–70, 91–5
    research 40–3, 116–19
    smoking 65–70
    stages v–vi, 5–10, 203
    STIs 110–19
    vaginal bleeding problems 153–61
exercise
    alcohol 75
    amenorrhoea 148, 150, 151
    menopause 165, 166
    obesity 55, 57, 60–2, 64
    polycystic ovarian syndrome 156
    women's health 76, 79
'expert patient' programme 23

Faculty of Family Planning and
        Reproductive Health Care 84
fallopian tubes (salpinges) 108, 124–5,
    134, 148

false-negative (-positive) results 63, 107,
    108, 114
family planning services
    confidentiality 50, 196
    contraception 39, 84, 93–4
    STIs 102
    teenagers 195–7
fat, in diet 55, 57, 60, 61
feedback
    360° feedback 17–19, 135, 180–1
    learning and service needs 3, 17–18,
        21–6, 30
    women's health and lifestyle 67, 77, 78,
        158
female condoms (Femidom) 85
fibroids 144
fitness to practise 2, 3
focus groups 26, 45
folic acid 123
follicle stimulating hormone (FSH) 123,
    126, 127, 151, 166, 170
force-field analysis 26–7
formication 164
Fraser guidelines
    consent and confidentiality 39, 47
    contraception 39, 82, 92, 95
    teenagers 189, 192
FSH *see* follicle stimulating hormone

galactorrhoea 137, 138
gall bladder disease 58
Gardnerella vaginosis 106 *see also* bacterial
    vaginosis
General Practice Assessment Questionnaire
    (GPAQ) 22
general practitioners *see* GPs
genital warts (HPV) 63, 103, 105, 110,
    112
genitourinary medicine (GUM) clinics 46,
    101–2, 109–12, 120
GGT (gamma glutamyl transpeptidase) 63
gonadotrophin releasing hormone (GnRH)
    agonists 145, 148, 166
gonorrhoea (GC) 103, 104, 107
*The Good Appraisal Toolkit* v
good medical practice (evidence cycles)
    70–6, 113–16, 131–3, 153–6,
    176–8
GPAQ (General Practice Assessment
    Questionnaire) 22

GPs (general practitioners)
   complaints 53
   consent and confidentiality 39, 46, 81
   contraception 81, 92, 94
   GUM clinics 101
   infertility 121
   learning and service needs 26
   patients' alcohol problems 62
   smoking cessation 68–9
   teenager-friendly consultations 189–91,
      196
guidelines
   complaints 53
   confidentiality 50
   contraception 86, 102, 197
   infertility 123, 125, 130, 133
   learning and service needs 20, 21, 26
   menopause 178, 183
   PDPs and appraisal 11
   STIs 109, 112, 118
   teenagers 191, 195
   vaginal bleeding problems 142, 155,
      159–61
   women's lifestyle 62, 67, 69–70, 72–3,
      75, 77–8
GUM clinics *see* genitourinary medicine clinics
gynaecologists 144, 145

hazards 27–8
HDL (high density lipoprotein) cholesterol
   59, 61
health and safety 9, 30, 69, 109, 114, 117
healthcare
   access and availability 26
   cost-effectiveness 32–3
   health promotion 67, 69, 76–9, 190,
      193
   inequalities 30, 83
   population health needs 30, 33, 193–5,
      199
Healthcare Commission 21, 68
heart disease
   lifestyle factors 55, 56, 58, 62
   menopause 167, 171
   obesity 57, 58, 61, 64
   smoking 55, 189
hepatitis 103, 105, 125
herpes 103, 107
high density lipoprotein (HDL) cholesterol
   59, 61

hirsutism 149, 151, 154
HIV *see* human immunodeficiency virus
homeopathy 166
hormone replacement therapy (HRT)
   advising on 166–9
   duration of treatment 169–72
   evidence cycles 176–8
hot flushes 151, 163–4, 166, 170, 172
HPV *see* human papilloma virus
hrqol (health-related quality of life) 32
HRT *see* hormone replacement therapy
Human Fertilisation and Embryology
      Authority (HFEA) 125
human immunodeficiency virus (HIV)
      103–6, 116, 118–19
human papilloma virus (HPV) 63, 103,
      105, 110, 112
hydrosalpinges 124–5, 134
hyperprolactinaemia 127, 151
hypertension 57–8, 60–1, 125, 152, 155
hypnotherapy 56
hypothalamic dysfunction 148, 150, 151,
      166
hysterectomy 106, 141, 144, 163, 168,
      170
hysterosalpingography 124, 134

ICSI *see* intracytoplasmic sperm injection
immunisations 45, 103
implants
   contraception 39, 87, 88, 97
   HRT 166, 168
impotence 126
infants 66–7, 83, 88, 104, 105
infection control 109
infertility
   age 122–3
   *Chlamydia* 104, 108, 193
   consultations 121
   infertility calculator 123
   male factors 124–31
   miscarriage 146
   polycystic ovarian syndrome 127, 133
   smoking 55
   tubal factors 124–5, 134
   vaginal bleeding problems 137–8, 145,
      153
informed consent *see also* consent
   emergency contraception 87
   evidence cycles 37–46

healthcare 35–6
learning needs 19
injections, contraceptive 39, 87, 88, 98
insulin 59, 127
insurance 36, 101
intermenstrual bleeding 142, 152–3, 168,
    172
intracytoplasmic sperm injection (ICSI)
    124–6
intrauterine device with copper (IUCD)
    87–9, 143
intrauterine devices (IUDs) 38–40, 86–9,
    96–7, 143, 147
intrauterine system with progesterone (IUS)
    89, 97–8, 141, 144, 170
irritable bowel syndrome 145, 147
IUCD *see* intrauterine device with copper
IUDs *see* intrauterine devices
IUS *see* intrauterine system with
    progesterone

journals 4, 24, 138

Knowledge and Skills Framework 24

laparoscopy 90, 144–5, 148
LDL (low density lipoprotein) cholesterol
    59
leaflets
    consent and confidentiality 42–3, 46
    contraception 83–7, 91, 93–4, 97
    menopause 167, 178
    STIs 104
    teenagers 42, 192
    vaginal bleeding problems 155, 157–8
learning *see also* learning needs
    complaints 51
    learning plans 33, 50, 75
    PDPs and appraisal 1–2, 4, 10–11
learning disabilities 44–6
learning needs *see also* learning
    assessment 18–19, 22
    audit 20–2
    evidence cycles 9–10, 203
    feedback 17–18, 22–3
    PDPs and appraisal 2, 5
    and service needs 26, 32–3
    standards and competence 15–16
    SWOT/SCOT analysis 23
    work environment 23–4

Levonelle/Levonelle-2 85, 87, 92, 95
levonorgestrel 141, 144
LH *see* luteinising hormone
lifelong learning v, 1–2, 5, 15, 203
lifestyle *see* women's health and lifestyle
lipids 59, 152
listeriosis 122
liver function 63, 86, 105, 165
LMP (last menstrual period) 86
Local Delivery Plans 33
local research ethics committees 36, 42–3
locums 31, 52–3, 91–5
long-acting contraception
    consent 38, 40
    consultations 84
    implants 39, 87, 88, 97
    injections 39, 87, 88, 98
    IUDs 38–40, 86–9, 96–7, 143, 147
    IUS 89, 97–8, 141, 144, 170
    patches 90
    sterilisation 89–90, 96–8
    vasectomy 89, 90, 97
low density lipoprotein (LDL) cholesterol
    59
lubricants 166, 172
lung cancer 55, 56
luteal phase 143, 164
luteinising hormone (LH) 123, 126, 127,
    151

mammograms 45, 76, 168
management 12, 116–19, 198–201
Masters' Frameworks 8
medroxyprogesterone acetate 88, 151
men's health
    infertility 124–31
    lifestyle 55, 57, 62
    STIs 103, 104
    vasectomy 89, 90, 97
MENCAP 45, 46
menopause
    age 163
    amenorrhoea 151, 152
    evidence cycles 173–84
    hot flushes 163–4, 166, 170, 172
    HRT
        advising on 166–9
        duration of treatment 169–72
        evidence cycles 176–8
    lifestyle advice 165–6

non-oestrogen treatments  171–2
osteoporosis  165, 168, 170–2
symptoms  164–7, 170
websites  185
menorrhagia  141–4
menstruation
amenorrhoea  137–8, 148–52, 172
contraception  81, 86–90
dysmenorrhoea  89, 141, 144–5
ectopic pregnancy  147
infertility  123, 127, 131, 137
menopause  163–6, 168, 172
menorrhagia  141–4
polycystic ovarian syndrome  127, 133,
154
STIs  103, 106
teenagers  188
mental health  12, 45, 46, 83, 189, 190
mentors  11, 18, 23, 27
metformin  127, 152
midstream urine (MSU)  107, 173–5
midwives  65, 146, 160
minority groups  25, 30
Mirena  89, 170
miscarriage
contraception  96
infertility  121, 123, 125
smoking  55
STIs  106
vaginal bleeding problems  145–7, 159–61
molluscum contagiosum  103–4
morbidity statistics  30, 55–9, 108, 194–5
mortality statistics  30, 55, 57, 59, 61, 83
MSU *see* midstream urine
*Mycoplasma genitalium*  104
myocardial infarction  57, 58

National electronic Library for Health  124
National Health Service *see* NHS
National Institute for Clinical Excellence
(NICE)  20, 33, 60, 71–3, 123, 130
National Prescribing Centre  v
National Service Frameworks  15, 20, 29,
33
needle-stick injuries  118
NHS (National Health Service)
consent  36, 39, 43
learning and service needs  23, 29
PDPs and appraisal  2–3, 9
smoking  55

NICE *see* National Institute for Clinical
Excellence
nicotine replacement therapy  56, 67, 78
NMC *see* Nursing and Midwifery Council
non-specific urethritis (NSU)  104, 113–16
noradrenaline reuptake inhibitors  60, 61
norethisterone  88, 172
Northern Ireland, health policies  47
NSU *see* non-specific urethritis
nucleic acid amplification tests  107, 108
*Nurse Prescribers' Formulary*  56
nurses
as advocates  44, 97, 132, 141
community psychiatric nurses  147, 151
complaints  52, 53
consent and confidentiality  39, 50
contraception  39, 86–7, 91–5
infertility  121–2
learning and service needs  15, 26
menopause clinics  182, 184
obesity therapy  59, 60, 62
patient group directions  87, 91–5
PDPs and appraisal  v–vi, 1, 3–5, 12
prescribing  37, 56, 71–2, 86–7, 169
smoking cessation  56, 68–9
specialists  7–8, 12, 15, 23, 94, 144
teenager-friendly consultations  39,
187–91
Nursing and Midwifery Council (NMC)
*Code of Professional Conduct*  1, 4–5, 35,
198
consent  35, 39
lifelong learning  1, 15
obesity  60
PDPs and appraisal  v, 2–5, 8, 11, 203

obesity
alcohol  62–3
body mass index  57, 58, 60, 72
contraception  84
diet  57, 59–61
drug therapy  59–61, 71–2
evidence cycles  70–3, 154–5
infertility  122, 124, 127
vaginal bleeding problems  142, 151,
154–5
women's lifestyle  55, 57–64, 78, 79
oestrogens
contraception  83, 90
menopause  164, 166–70, 172

vaginal bleeding problems  142, 145,
     151, 152
oral contraception (pill)
     contraceptive advice  29, 81–3, 85, 90,
          93, 98
     teenagers  189
     vaginal bleeding problems  152–3, 156,
          158
orlistat (Xenical)  60, 61, 72–3
osteoporosis  77, 165, 168, 170–2
ovaries *see also* ovulation; polycystic ovarian
          syndrome
     ectopic pregnancy  147
     infertility  127
     menopause  163, 166, 172
     ovarian cancer  58, 127, 172
     vaginal bleeding problems  145, 151
overweight  57, 60, 62, 72, 96 *see also*
          obesity
ovulation  87, 122–3, 127, 148–9, 164 *see
          also* ovaries
oxytetracycline  113, 115–16

pain
     dyspareunia  106, 142, 169, 170
     STIs  103, 104, 108
     vaginal bleeding problems  89, 144–5,
          147–8, 151
     vasectomy  90
parental consent  39, 47, 82, 84, 192
patches, contraceptive  90
patient group directions (PGDs)  86–7,
          92–4
patients
     complaints  51–4
     consent and confidentiality  37–43,
          46–7, 49
     evidence cycles
          consent  37–40
          contraception  91–8
          health promotion  76–9
          infertility  134–6
          menopause  176–81
          obesity  72–3
          STIs  110–12
          teenagers  193–5
          vaginal bleeding problems  156–8
     learning and service needs  15–16, 19,
          22–3, 25–6, 30, 33
     PDPs and appraisal  9, 11, 12

rights  19–20, 41, 46, 77, 111, 191
safety  9, 30, 69, 109, 114, 117
satisfaction surveys
     consent  39–43
     contraception  93–4, 97–8
     lifestyle  66–7, 72–3, 75
     service needs  11, 22–3
PCOs *see* primary care organisations
PCOS *see* polycystic ovarian syndrome
PCTs *see* primary care trusts
PDPs *see* personal development plans
peer review  21, 27, 42, 43, 53, 78
pelvic examinations  46, 149
pelvic inflammatory disease (PID)  106,
          111, 124, 145, 147
Pendleton model of feedback  17
performance assessment  2–5, 16–18,
          20–1, 29, 203
perimenopause  163, 166, 185
periods *see* menstruation
personal development plans (PDPs)
     alcohol  75
     appraisal  v–vi, 2–4, 11, 203
     learning and service needs  16, 33
     lifelong learning  1–2, 5
personal professional profile (PPP)  3, 4
PGDs *see* patient group directions
pharmacists  50, 85, 195, 197
phenytoin  63, 86
physical examinations
     breasts  53, 77, 149, 150, 168
     contraception  83
     pelvic  46, 149
phytoestrogens  166
PID *see* pelvic inflammatory disease
the pill *see* oral contraception
polycystic ovarian syndrome (PCOS)  127,
          133, 142, 150–2, 154–6
polyps  152
POP (progestogen-only pill)  85, 96
population health needs  30, 33, 193–5,
          199
portfolios
     evidence cycles  6, 8, 203
     learning and service needs  9, 15, 16,
          22, 78
     PDPs and appraisal  v, 1–5, 10–12
postcoital bleeding  142, 152–3, 156–7,
          172
postmenopause  62, 163, 170, 172

postnatal depression  83
post-registration  1–5, 11
post-registration education and practice (PREP)  1, 3–5
PPP *see* personal professional profile
practitioner with special interest (PwSI)  12
pregnancy
    consent and confidentiality  38, 40, 49, 197
    contraception  38, 40, 81, 85, 87–8, 199
    ectopic pregnancy  147–8
    infertility  121–6
    menopause  163
    miscarriage  96, 106, 145–7, 159–61
    multiple pregnancies  127
    service needs  21, 30
    smoking  55, 65–7
    STIs  105, 106, 113–16
    teenagers  81–4, 188, 190, 192–4, 197, 199–200
    terminations  38, 49, 81, 147, 197, 199
    vaginal bleeding problems  145–51
premature birth  55, 88, 106
premature menopause  151, 163, 165–6, 168, 171–2
premenstrual symptoms  88, 142, 163, 170
PREP *see* post-registration education and practice
prescribing
    consent and confidentiality  37
    emergency contraception  86–7
    HRT  169
    National Prescribing Centre  v
    obesity drug therapy  60, 71–2
    smoking cessation  56
    STIs  113–16
primary amenorrhoea  149–50
primary care organisations (PCOs)
    alcohol  62
    complaints  54
    contraception  94, 97–8, 200
    evidence cycles  42, 43, 53, 94
    learning and service needs  21, 30, 33
    menopause  182–3
    PDPs and appraisal  2, 9, 12
    STIs  109, 118
    teenagers  200
primary care trusts (PCTs)  18, 21, 68, 70, 93

privacy  52, 53, 196
probity  68–70, 91–5
Prodigy  149
progesterone  123, 126, 146, 164, 166–7
progestogens
    emergency contraception  85, 94
    long-acting contraception  88, 143
    menopause  168–70, 172
    progestogen-only pill  85, 96
    side-effects  85–8
    vaginal bleeding problems  143, 145, 150–2
prolactin  127, 148, 150–2
protocols *see* guidelines
psychological conditions  56, 61, 62, 151, 163–5, 189–90
puberty  148, 149
public health data  30, 194–5, 199–200
PwSI *see* practitioner with special interest

quality assessment  2, 31–2, 203
questionnaires
    alcohol  63, 75
    evidence cycles  41, 75, 116, 118, 195
    learning and service needs  17, 22–3

rape  47
RCOG *see* Royal College of Obstetricians and Gynaecologists
recurrent miscarriage  146, 159–61
Reductil (sibutramine)  60, 61, 72
referrals
    consent  36, 49
    menopause  172, 176–8
    service needs  26, 30
    STIs  111
reflective diaries
    contraception  94, 97–8
    infertility  136
    menopause  180
    STIs  111–12
    vaginal bleeding problems  155, 158
    women's lifestyle  72
reflective writing  5, 11, 24, 203
registration  1–5, 11, 203
research
    ethics  36, 42–3
    evidence cycles  6, 40–3, 116–19
    miscarriage  146

portfolios  11, 12
service needs  29
resources  8, 15, 23, 25
risk assessment
    alcohol  63
    confidentiality and consent  36, 47
    contraception  85
    HRT  167, 170–1
    obesity  57, 58
    screening tests  77–8
    service needs  27–8
    smoking  55–6, 66–7
    STIs  103, 117
    teenagers  83, 192–3
roles/responsibilities
    competence  7
    contraception  93, 95–8
    learning and service needs  15, 24, 32
    PDPs and appraisal  v, 9, 10
    role play  136, 180
    teamworking  44, 68–70
Royal College of Nursing  168
Royal College of Obstetricians and
        Gynaecologists (RCOG)  142–3,
        145, 146
Royal College of Physicians  171
rubella  123, 126

safety  9, 30, 69, 109, 114, 117
salpinges (fallopian tubes)  108, 124–5,
        134, 148
schools  94–5, 189–90, 192, 197
SCOT analysis (strengths, challenges,
        opportunities and threats)  23, 75–6
Scotland, health policies  20, 47, 87, 120
Scottish Intercollegiate Guidelines Network
        (SIGN)  20, 120
screening tests *see also* cervical smears
    alcohol  74
    consent  45
    STIs  87, 102, 104, 107–9, 116–19
    teenagers  188
    'well woman' checks  55, 63–4, 76–9
secondary amenorrhoea  150–2
secondary sexual characteristics  149–50
selective oestrogen receptor modulators
        (SERMs)  171–2
self-assessment
    evidence cycles  45, 66, 111, 135
    learning needs  11, 18–19, 24

semen analysis  123, 124–6, 128–31
sequential therapy (HRT)  167, 169–70,
        172, 176–8
SERMs *see* selective oestrogen receptor
        modulators
serotonin reuptake inhibitors (SSRIs)  60,
        61, 172
service needs
    cost-effectiveness  32–3
    evaluation  28–9
    feedback  25–6
    force-field analysis  26–7
    and learning needs  15–17
    legislation  30
    PDPs and appraisal  2, 9–10, 203
    risk assessment  27–8
    setting priorities  25, 33
sex hormone binding globulin (SHBG)  127,
        169
sexual abuse  47, 83
sexual health
    contraception  81, 94
    menopause  182
    STIs  101–3, 109, 116
    teenagers  188–9, 198–201
    women's lifestyle  63–4
*Sexual Health Matters in Primary Care*  109
sexual intercourse *see also* contraception;
        sexually transmitted infections;
        unprotected sexual intercourse
    consent and confidentiality  38, 47
    infertility  122
    pain  106, 142, 169, 170
    STIs  102–3, 105–7
    teenagers  82–3, 191
    vaginal dryness  164, 166
sexually transmitted infections (STIs)
    bacterial vaginosis  104, 106, 107
    *Chlamydia*  103–4, 107, 116–19, 193
    condoms  84–5, 103, 188
    genital warts (HPV)  63, 103, 105, 110,
        112
    gonorrhoea  103, 104, 107
    GUM clinics  46, 101–3, 109–12, 120
    hepatitis  103, 105, 125
    herpes  103, 107
    HIV  103–6, 116, 118–19
    infertility  104, 193
    non-specific urethritis  104, 113–16
    screening tests  63, 107, 116–19

syphilis 103, 105
teenagers 82, 188–90, 193, 194
thrush 104, 106, 107
trichomonas 105, 107
SHBG *see* sex hormone binding globulin
sibutramine (Reductil) 60, 61, 72
side-effects
    anti-obesity therapy 60–1, 72
    consent 42
    contraception 85–8
    HRT 169
    significant event audit 21
SIGN *see* Scottish Intercollegiate Guidelines
        Network
significant event audit
    contraception 97–8, 200
    evidence cycles 45, 52–3, 66, 78, 155
    learning and service needs 21–2, 28
    STIs 111, 115
skin conditions 105, 189–90 *see also* acne
sleep disturbance 56, 62, 74, 76, 164
smears *see* cervical smears
smoking
    alcohol 75, 76
    amenorrhoea 150
    contraception 38, 84, 85, 88, 96
    infertility 123
    menopause 165, 166
    obesity 57, 64
    teenagers 83, 188–90, 193
    women's lifestyle 55–6, 65–70, 76, 79
Social Exclusion Unit 82
sperm counts 124–31, 134
St John's Wort 167
sterilisation 89–90, 96–8
STIs *see* sexually transmitted infections
streptococcus 103
stress 148, 150, 164–6
stroke 58, 62, 78, 167
students 42, 49–50, 183, 197
substance misuse 30, 46, 75, 83, 193
supervision 8, 24, 94, 182
swabs 39, 104, 106–7, 108, 113
SWOT analysis (strengths, weaknesses,
        opportunities and threats) 23, 24,
        175
syphilis 103, 105

tamoxifen 142, 171
Tanner's stages of puberty 149

teaching and training
    consent 36
    evidence cycles
        confidentiality 48–50
        contraception 92
        infertility 136–8, 159–61
        menopause 181–4
        teenagers 193–8
        training needs 94, 116–19
    learning and service needs 12, 17, 31,
        33, 75, 182–4
teamwork 26, 30, 36, 68–70, 75, 115
teenagers
    confidentiality 46–7, 187, 196–8
    consent 39, 41–3, 46–7, 49–50
    consultations 189–91
    contraception
        consent and confidentiality 39,
            49–50
        emergency contraception 91–5
        teenage pregnancy 81–4
        teenager-friendly services 191,
            196–201
    evidence cycles 91–5
    lifestyle advice 189–91
    nurses 187–8
    service needs 30, 191–2
    sexual health 104, 188–9
termination of pregnancy 38, 49, 81, 147,
        197, 199
testicles 126, 127
testosterone 127, 151
thrombosis 58, 84, 90, 167–9, 171–2
thrush 104, 106, 107
thyroid function 127, 142, 149–51, 166
tibolone 167, 169
toxoplasmosis 122
tracer criteria 21
training *see* teaching and training
tranexamic acid 21, 143
transitional zone 64, 107
trichomonas vaginalis 105, 107
triglycerides 59, 61
TSH (thyroid stimulating hormone) 127
Turner's syndrome 148, 149

UKCC (United Kingdom Central Council)
        3
ultrasound scans 145, 148, 151, 156
universities 8, 11, 12, 183–4

unprotected sexual intercourse (UPSI)
    consent and confidentiality  38, 47
    emergency contraception  38, 40, 81,
        85–7, 89, 91–5
    teenagers  81, 83, 191
*Ureaplasma urealyticum*  104
urethritis  104, 113–16
urine tests  107, 108, 113, 147
urogenital conditions  170, 173–5
uterus
    infertility  124
    STIs  102, 108
    vaginal bleeding  141–2, 144, 148, 151

vaginal bleeding problems
    amenorrhoea  137–8, 148–52, 172
    consent  46
    dysmenorrhoea  89, 141, 144–5
    ectopic pregnancy  104, 108, 147–8
    endometriosis  122, 144–5
    intermenstrual bleeding  142, 152–3,
        168, 172
    menopause  168–9, 172, 176, 178
    menorrhagia  141–4
    miscarriage  145–7, 159–61
    polycystic ovarian syndrome  150–2,
        154–6
    postcoital bleeding  142, 152–3, 156–7,
        172
    STIs  103
vaginal dryness  164, 169, 172
varicocele  126
vas deferens  126
vasectomy  89, 90, 97
venous thrombosis  58, 84, 167, 171–2

videotapes  11, 24, 39, 50, 167
vitamin D  150, 165, 168, 171

Wales, health policies  21, 47, 63, 87
warfarin  166
warts, genital (HPV)  63, 103, 105, 110,
        112
weight gain/loss
    contraceptive injections  88
    HIV  105
    infertility  122–4, 127
    menopause  165, 166
    obesity  57–61, 70–3
    vaginal bleeding problems  148–52,
        154–6
'well woman' checks  55, 63, 76–9, 154
WHO *see* World Health Organization
withdrawal bleeding  151, 153, 172
women's health and lifestyle *see also* diet
    alcohol  55, 62–3, 73–6, 165–6
    exercise  62, 75, 165
    obesity  57–64, 70–3
    sexual health  63–4
    smoking  55–6, 65–70
    'well woman' checks  55, 63–4, 76–9
workshops
    alcohol  75
    menopause  183
    smoking  70
    STIs  112, 118
    teenagers  193, 197, 200
World Health Organization (WHO)  84,
        125, 130

Xenical (orlistat)  60, 61, 72–3